Dementia
Beyond
Drugs

Dementia Beyond Drugs

CHANGING THE CULTURE OF CARE

by G. ALLEN POWER, M.D., FACP

Foreword by William H. Thomas, M.D.

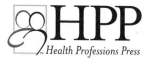
Health Professions Press

Baltimore • London • Sydney

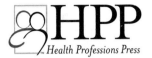

Health Professions Press, Inc.
Post Office Box 10624
Baltimore, Maryland 21285-0624

www.healthpropress.com

Interior and cover designs by Mindy Dunn.
Typeset by Karen Wenk.
Manufactured in the United States of America by Versa Press, East Peoria, Illinois.

The names of the people with dementia in this book have been changed to respect their privacy.

The following materials are reproduced by permission of Jessica Kingsley Publishers: The extracts on pages 83, 113, 137, 138, 178, 192, and 242 are from *Dancing with Dementia: My Story of Living Positively with Dementia*, by Christine Bryden. Copyright (c) 2005 by Christine Bryden. The extract on pages 145–146 is from *Person-Centred Dementia Care: Making Services Better*, by Dawn Brooker. Copyright © 2007 by Dawn Brooker.

Library of Congress Cataloging-in-Publication Data

Power, G. Allen.
  Dementia beyond drugs : changing the culture of care / G. Allen Power.
      p. ; cm.
  Includes bibliographical references and index.
  ISBN 978-1-932529-56-2 (pbk.)
  1. Dementia—Patients—Care. 2. Dementia—Treatment. I. Title.
  [DNLM: 1. Dementia—therapy. 2. Aged. 3. Attitude of Health Personnel.
  4. Dementia—psychology. 5. Homes for the Aged. 6. Nursing Homes. WM 220 P887d 2010]
  RC521.P69 2010
  616.8′3—dc22   2009048654

British Library Cataloguing in Publication data are available from the British Library.

This book is dedicated to my greatest teachers—the people I have known and cared for who have lived with dementia.

"When the facts change, I change my mind. What do you do, sir?"
—John Maynard Keynes

CONTENTS

FOREWORD

Dr. Al Power is an artist. He is an established singer–songwriter with multiple albums, and his music speaks to the heart of life and living. I mention this not because I am urging you to go and buy his albums, but because an artist's perspective, overlaid on his wealth of clinical experience with dementia, animates so much of what is important about this book.

Conventional wisdom, if you can call it that, holds that dementia represents a peculiar, deadly, and completely irredeemable kind of decline. It is the ultimate down escalator—destination oblivion. This pervasive biomedical mindset that focuses only on physical and cognitive decline shapes the views of doctors, patients, and families alike. The daughter of a woman living with dementia wrote the following on her Web blog:

> We took [Mom] to several doctors, trying desperately to reverse or at least slow down her physical and mental deterioration. The doctors were compassionate, but had very little help. There were medications to treat her symptoms, but nothing that made any real difference. Eventually trips to the doctor just became too difficult for her. We couldn't continue to put her through the ordeal of another ride on the nursing home van, and sitting in a doctor's lobby when she couldn't even hold herself upright in her wheelchair. It was too hard. (Retrieved November 30, 2009, from http://deborahfoster.wordpress.com/the-dementia-decline-continues-sigh/.)

She tells a similar tale to the ones I heard from many kind and loving adult children I worked with during my years in practice. Help for a loved one living with dementia is equated simply and directly with diagnosis and medical treatment. Indeed, there are powerful forces inside the medical profession and the medical–industrial complex that are well served by perpetuating this false equivalence between care and treatment. In fact, the words *care* and *treatment* have been pushed and pulled so far from their original meanings it is worth revisiting them.

The most common and useful definition of *care* I know goes like this: "Care means helping a person or relationship to grow." We care for our children because we want to see them grow. People care for a marriage when they want their relationship with a spouse to deepen, to strengthen, to grow. Healthy growth is always an organic multifaceted process. Growth releases latent potential, which is why genuine growth so often surprises us.

Treatment, in particular medical treatment, reduces complex phenomena to simple chains of cause and effect. Conventional medicine (also known as allopathic medicine) is based on the idea that we should counteract one condition with a pill that causes the opposite condition. This simple idea lies behind almost all of the most powerful healing drugs and therapies available to us today.

Although the terms *care* and *treatment* are often, and thoughtlessly, used interchangeably, they offer radically divergent paths to health and happiness. The tension between medical treatment and genuine human caring erupts into the open when they are applied to the experiences of people living with dementia.

As of this writing, there is no simple, well-tolerated medication capable of "curing" dementia. I am an optimist by nature, but, even so, I would be willing to bet there will *never* be a simple, well-tolerated medical cure for dementia. Why not? The human brain is an astonishingly complicated organ and its workings are vastly more complicated than the simple chains of cause and effect on which most medical treatments rely.

Nonmedical approaches to the well-being of people living with dementia can go far beyond anything any pill has to offer. Consider this sketch of an organic, growth-oriented approach to the experience of people living with dementia in Australia:

> A group of mothers and children meet regularly for playgroup with residents at a dementia specific hostel in Perth, Western Australia. "Even after initial visits we could see beautiful friendships beginning to emerge between the residents, mothers and children." . . . The playgroup offers (people living with dementia) an outlet to express their love for others. When residents are with the children, they appear more responsive and happier. . . .
>
> Involvement in the intergenerational program at the facility has provided us with better understanding and the realisation that often the best therapy is to provide opportunities for happiness and increased meaning in the lives of residents. [Emphasis added] (Retrieved November 30, 2009, from http://www.dementiacareaustralia.com/index/php/ community/bridging-the-generation-gap-with-love.html)

The intergenerational program at this facility was under the guidance of Hilary Lee, and drew inspiration from Jane Verity's Spark of Life approach that she was currently researching. Jane's ideas are presented in this book alongside those of similar innovators in dementia care. Her explorations on the frontier of dementia challenge the assumption that groundbreaking research must take place in sterile industrial laboratories. In truth, the breakthroughs we need most, the research that can lead us to synthesize the best of medical and nonmedical approaches, can take place anywhere and anytime we encounter people living with dementia and the people who love and care for them.

Which brings me back to art. An artist must be comfortable with complexity, with nuance, with uncertainty. The magic of art lies in the artist's ability to integrate scattered bits of color, light, sound, and symbols into enduring expressions of truth and beauty. I see this book as a work of art because it creates a new space within a field that has long been constrained by narrow mechanistic and biomedical interpretations of the dementia experience. The time is right for a geriatrician–humanitarian–singer–songwriter–author to redraw the boundaries of what is possible. Our field is in the early years of a transformation that will remake aging-related organizations' policies, structures, and financing. If we are fortunate, *Dementia Beyond Drugs* will earn a place as a foundational text for those who are committed to re-imagining the services we provide people living with dementia.

William H. Thomas, M.D.
Founder, The Eden Alternative

ACKNOWLEDGMENTS

This book has been a long time in the making and it would be impossible to list all of the people who have enriched my journey. Nevertheless, I could not pass this opportunity to thank several people for their contributions to this project, and to the ideas that led me down this path.

I am indebted to Mary Magnus, publications director for Health Professions Press, for embracing a book that challenges much of the prevailing wisdom on dementia. Mary and her staff have been unflagging in their support for this project. Cecilia González has patiently guided me through the production process and answered my myriad questions each step of the way. Thanks also to Kristi Maxwell for her marketing and promotional efforts. My thanks as well to Diane Ersepke for her thoughtful copyediting and to Mindy Dunn for her striking book design.

There are no words adequate to thank Bill and Jude Thomas, founders of the Eden Alternative, for their vision, passion, friendship, guidance, and support. They have literally changed my life and my career.

I am also grateful for the support of the Eden Alternative family, who work tirelessly to create a life worth living for our elders and those who care for them. I cannot begin to thank all of the people who have contributed to my understanding of this transformational movement. I will mention a few, however, who have directly educated me on culture change or provided resources for the ideas expressed in this book: Carol Ende, Susan Berta, Nancy Fox, Denise Hyde, Laura Beck, Emi Kiyota, Hilary Lee, Christa Monkhouse, Vicki Rosebrook, Dorene Spies, and Jane Verity.

I am proud to be a member of the community of St. John's Home, and I hope this book will serve as a token of my appreciation for the friendship and support I have received over the past decade. Thanks in particular to Charlie Runyon and Veronica Barber for giving me the resources and support to pursue this path, to my medical colleagues past and present for inspiring and challenging me, and to all of my co-workers who strive every day to create a place of caring and compassion for all.

Heartfelt thanks to friends and colleagues who have read parts of this manuscript at various stages and provided valuable feedback: Mimi

Bommelje, Dr. William Hall, Eileen Hayes-Power, Dr. Emi Kiyota, Cathi Laturi, Dr. Robert McCann, Christa Monkhouse, Ora Power, Dr. Timothy Quill, Dr. William Thomas, Alan Whitney, Carter Catlett Williams, and Dr. T. Franklin Williams.

I am also grateful to Beth Baker, Andrea Ruggieri, and Joe LaMay for technical support along the way.

My work stands firmly on the shoulders of many others who have espoused a more humanistic approach to the care of those who live with dementia. Many of them are mentioned in these pages, and I am grateful to them for sharing their ideas with me and with the world.

A very satisfied thank you to the fine folks at Café Cibon, who have provided so much of the "fuel" for the writing of this book over the past few years.

Finally, much love and appreciation to my family—my wife Eileen and my children Ian and Caitlin—for their support every step of the way.

Simone's Story

THIS IS A STORY OF FAILURE. I realize that is not the usual way to start a book like this, but the story typifies the experiences of many who care for people with dementia. There are no bad guys in this story; all are good, caring people who try their best to provide compassionate care, but fall short nonetheless.

Stories are important when discussing different approaches to care, because they bring an essential humanity to the issues at hand. This is where our current system has gone astray; we have lost the humanity in our biomedical approach to caring for people with dementia. This is the story of Simone:

> Simone came to live at the nursing home at the age of 92. A former bookkeeper, she had divorced many years earlier and had no children. Her only relatives were a sister, two nephews, and their families. She worked well beyond the traditional retirement age and also helped watch her nephews' children when they were young.
>
> Simone lived in an apartment complex but developed signs of dementia. She began to get lost in the complex and became more confused and unable to manage alone. She was put on the waiting list for an assisted living apartment but ended up in the

hospital with what appeared to be a sudden worsening of her confusion. Blood tests and X rays were ordered and a few doses of antibiotics were given, but no obvious cause was found outside of her probable dementia. It was decided that she needed to be in a nursing home.

During her hospital stay, Simone was noted to be "belligerent," resisting examinations and treatments, and pulling out her IV lines. She was given an antipsychotic medication, as is commonly done for such people with dementia. When she arrived at our door, she was barely arousable, due to a combination of sedating medication and lack of sleep.

Later, when she was better rested, Simone was pleasant but had little understanding of her situation, and she was unable to give me any medical history. The antipsychotic medication was slowly withdrawn, and she became more alert and began to walk independently again. Unfortunately, as she became more aware of her surroundings, her distress increased as well.

What followed was a very stormy 7 months. Simone's mood fluctuated, often with little warning. She could be friendly and affectionate one moment, and then suddenly she could become angry—shouting, resisting attempts at personal care, or even throwing objects around the room. During these episodes, the nurses and aides were often unable to approach her and had to leave her alone until she felt calmer.

At one point, Simone had to be moved from her double room to a private room down the hall. She had a roommate who couldn't speak and was totally dependent for care due to advanced Alzheimer's disease. Simone would try to lift her out of her chair or spoon-feed her as if she were an infant. She still wanted to be a caregiver but had no safe outlet for doing so.

During these months, several medications were tried without benefit. Simone acted depressed at times, but antidepressant medication didn't seem to help. At times she seemed to be in pain, but there was no consistent benefit to pain medication. A trial of the seizure medication valproic acid (often used for behavioral symptoms) was also fruitless, and she would not take most doses when offered.

We held many meetings and brainstorming sessions trying to find a better approach. Her niece said that meaningful work was always very important to Simone, so we looked for ways to occupy her with simple tasks, such as sorting papers or folding washcloths. Some days this worked, but on others she could not attend to the activity.

There was another story evolving at the same time, however, and that was my own. This created a dynamic that, in many ways, was the motivation for this book. Allow me to back up and interject a bit of my own history.

I entered medical school in the late 1970s. Inspired by our family doctor, Edwin Olsan, I planned a career as a general internist. After completing a residency and chief residency in internal medicine, I entered private practice in 1984.

I enjoyed the world of private practice, but it was an all-consuming lifestyle. I wasn't seeing enough of my family or engaging in the other pursuits, such as music, that had provided balance in my life. One day, after nearly 7 years of practice, I was in the doctors' lounge at the local hospital, Rochester General, and noticed an ad for a physician to fill a vacancy at a nearby nursing home.

Before that day, the idea of working full time in a nursing home was one I never would have considered, even for a moment. "Too depressing," I would have said. But something made me decide to investigate.

Dr. Jim Wood was a former internist who had left practice himself after 7 years to become the medical director at the home. I went to talk to him about the job, and I liked what I saw. The idea of caring for people in their own "home" was appealing to me, as house calls had become nearly impossible in my busy private practice.

I was about to make the first of a series of very unorthodox decisions in my life. It wasn't always this way for me; I was quiet and introspective by nature, with very middle-of-the-road attitudes about many social and political issues. I sought counsel with Rochester General's chief of medicine, Dr. William Hall (who was making his own mark in shifting from pulmonary medicine to geriatrics).

Bill Hall's advice was simple: "Sure. Go for it. There's no downside. You're a good doctor—if it doesn't work out, you can hang out another shingle and your patients will come right back!"

Other colleagues were less understanding. This was at a time when the prevailing wisdom was that people only worked in nursing homes when they couldn't make it anywhere else. Some people would approach me in the hospital hallways and give me a sympathetic nod, or place a hand on my shoulder and say, "How's it going, Al? Everything okay?" as if I had a drug problem, or maybe had run afoul of the Department of Health. Why else would a "rising star" of private practice do such a thing?

I had many older patients in my practice, but no special interest or expertise in the care of older adults. Regardless, I took the job and quickly began to love my work. The same colleagues came up to me in the hospital a year later and said, "Gee, Al, you seem to be the happiest person around here. I wish I had the guts to do what you did!"

And so it went for over 6 years. We had a great nursing home and a crack medical team. We gave the best care on the planet. So I thought.

My world started to change irreversibly in late 1997. One of our social workers, Ann Pennell, told me about a nursing home in central New York that allowed dogs, cats, and birds to live there, and created a much warmer environment. As with most people, this rather simplistic description was how we first learned about a new movement called the Eden Alternative™.

Ann arranged for a woman named Susan Berta to come to our nursing home and tell the staff all about the movement. Susan, a former director of nursing for many years, was in the process of leaving her nursing home career to teach about the Eden Alternative on a full-time basis. I went to the talk, expecting to learn the nuts and bolts of how to bring animals into a nursing home without spreading infections. What I got instead was an eye-opening glance into a new philosophy of care.

After the meeting, I asked Susan for the phone number of Dr. William Thomas, the founder of the Eden Alternative. The following February, I toured four Eden homes across the state, and then followed Bill Thomas around for three frenetic days, running back and forth from his office to the nursing home. We went to a small-town public library one evening, where I watched him speak to a handful of locals about this fledgling movement to create a new world of elder care. It was very much a grassroots process in those days.

In September 1998, I attended a 4-day seminar taught by Bill and his wife, Jude Meyers-Thomas, and I became a Certified Eden Associate. It was a life-changing event.

When I returned to my job the following week, I felt like Dorothy did in *The Wizard of Oz,* when she opened the door of her farmhouse and the film went from black-and-white to Technicolor. I saw things I had never noticed in my 7 years of nursing home practice. Many things I thought I had done well now became shortcomings in my mind. I saw the plagues of institutionalization—loneliness, helplessness, and boredom—on the faces of the elders, and I felt their despair. They hadn't changed, but I saw them like never before. I became intent on changing the system. I began to speak fanatically about it—Eden can do that to a person.

I wanted our home to embark on the Eden Alternative pathway as quickly as possible. I was soon disappointed that not everyone shared my sense of urgency. There were too many other irons in the fire. Maybe in a couple of years. Maybe.

Patience was never my strong suit. I was so committed to this new path that "maybe" didn't cut it, so I decided to go out and find a place that was looking for a new direction. I have been told that if you put your intentions out to the world, the universe seems to send the right people to help. I'm not sure if it's all that mystical, but nevertheless I gave 6 months' notice and started visiting other nursing homes around town to see where I might generate some excitement about the Eden Alternative. This was not an easy job, because most homes are not able to employ doctors full time, let alone willing to embark on a path to transform their whole model of care.

After several months, I had pieced together a job proposal with a local health system that would have me working at several nursing homes and a hospital, and I almost convinced myself I could get something started this way. In the summer of 1999, a few days before I was to sign the contract, Rochester hosted the first national gathering of the Pioneer Network (an organization that had been created the previous year to enable innovators in elder care to share their stories and best practices). I ran into Dr. Marie Aydelotte, the medical director of St. John's Home, and she asked me if I wanted to apply for a position on their staff. After some cajoling, I agreed to come take a tour, fully expecting to turn her down after a polite inquiry. What I saw was a warm environment with many caring employees who seemed open to new ideas. I also met the administrator, Charlie Runyon. At the time, Charlie was not happy with the trends in long-term care, and he was looking for a new direction. He was also born and raised in Bill Thomas's hometown of Sherburne, New York, and there I was, talking about the Eden Alternative. Maybe there's something to this synchronicity after all.

To make a long story short, I took the job at St. John's Home, and I have been there for 10 years. We are now an Eden Alternative home, and we are moving slowly on our transformational journey, as large homes must. We have had many great accomplishments, some of which I will share in this book. During this time, I have become close to Bill and Jude Thomas and have become active in the Eden Alternative as a Mentor and Educator. My own ideas have been evolving quickly as well.

As I began to articulate the problems with the traditional nursing home model, I began to notice how the institutional approach to dementia created much of the distress seen in people with the illness. I also became frustrated at the poor results I was getting when using

~~medications to treat the behavioral expressions of dementia.~~ My experiences were telling me things that the medical journals were not. New reports of drug side effects added a worrisome dimension to their use as well.

~~I began giving lectures about addressing the behavioral symptoms~~ ~~of dementia without using drugs.~~ Sometimes my ideas worked well, but other times they fell short. ~~My experiences in caring for~~ Simone and ~~others like her have helped me stop, look at my ideas, and reorganize~~ ~~them in order to gain a better perspective about what is truly needed to~~ ~~unmedicate people with dementia and reconnect them with life.~~ Unfortunately, Simone didn't have a chance to benefit. The rest of her story is one that plays out again and again in people with advancing dementia.

> Much of the difficulty in caring for Simone came from the extreme unpredictability of her symptoms. Much difficulty also came from the internal tug-of-war between many caring people who were approaching the problem from different perspectives. Some of the staff wanted more medication, and other medications were tried, but her frequent refusal of pills made it difficult for us to reach conclusions. Often she would be very lethargic. Was it the pill or the fact that she had been awake most of the night before? For my part, I wanted more detective work to find clues to her unmet needs. We didn't always communicate well; I now see that I was so invested in moving innovation forward that I left many others behind. I knew from my Eden training that Simone had spiritual and existential needs that were not being met. We were not yet evolved to a place where we had the resources and organizational structure to effectively meet those needs.
>
> There were some positive moments. The nurses summoned me on one particularly difficult Friday afternoon. Simone was angrily fussing with a pile of linen on a cart and wouldn't let anyone near her to redirect her. Over the next half hour, I was able to intervene in a way that calmed her greatly and left her smiling and relaxed. (I will describe this intervention in detail later in the book.) Her pleasant demeanor lasted about 6 hours, although she became agitated once again at bedtime. I had been able to find important clues to connecting with Simone, but some staff members were discouraged that the intervention was short-lived, and they didn't feel they had time or resources to repeatedly engage her as I had. At that stage in our organizational journey, they were right.
>
> There was never a time over those 7 months when one could say that things went smoothly for Simone or for her care

staff. She was one of the toughest cases we had ever had. She eventually became aggressive toward another resident of the home, which forced our hand. We either had to medicate her or send her to an acute hospital, where she would certainly be restrained and sedated.

We started her on the antipsychotic drug olanzapine. This was chosen because it came in a form that dissolved under the tongue, which was much more reliable than getting her to swallow a pill or accept an injection. The dose (5 milligrams a day with an additional 2.5 milligrams if needed) was the lowest available and well in line with current prescribing guidelines.

Over the next three days, Simone fell four times. She didn't suffer any injury, but she never walked again. She was lethargic at times and needed more help with meals. She couldn't express herself as clearly and seemed to have episodes of "spacing out" when I spoke to her. Still, there were days when she continued to resist and fight back when her caregivers approached. Her oral intake and overall alertness declined. We had been following a "hospice" approach, due to her advanced dementia and her longstanding refusal of pills and blood tests. In keeping with that philosophy, aggressive measures were not taken to force-feed her.

One could easily say that Simone's severe dementia was the ultimate cause of her decline. And yet, until the day she started the olanzapine, she was able to walk (even run down the hall), communicate on some level, and eat independently. Six weeks later, Simone was dead.

The medication successfully prevented any further aggression toward other elders, at least in part because she could no longer walk. But it did not make her feel relaxed and comfortable in her surroundings. It did not stop her from resisting personal care. It did not improve her engagement with others or overall well-being. And it did not relieve her suffering; even when she was unable to speak, you could see that in her eyes.

We all tried our very best to help Simone. Her medication was completely in accordance with current guidelines. This is not an uncommon outcome in people with advancing dementia. How often are we forced to choose between sedating people and allowing them to be a potential danger to themselves or others?

There is a third option, one that addresses these symptoms effectively without using sedating medications. This choice is not readily available to most of us today because it requires us to drastically change the way we think and act in caring for people with dementia. We can improve the lives of some people quickly, but others, like Simone, require a much deeper *transformation* of the care environment before any real progress can be made. We need to start as soon as possible.

In spite of disappointments such as Simone's case, we have also seen many successes at St. John's, and our overall use of sedating medication is much lower than what is seen in most nursing homes. In recent years, I have traveled around the country, crossed the Atlantic and Pacific, hearing the tales of others who have succeeded as well. But now I better understand the process of change.

It is not enough simply to give advice on "managing behavioral symptoms." We cannot truly enrich the lives of people with dementia until we change many of our own fundamental beliefs about this condition and about elder care in general. My paths as a doctor and an Eden Alternative Educator are finally coming together in the writing of this book.

In these pages, I will share some remarkable stories of caring for people who live with dementia. Together with the reader I hope to create a pathway to a world in which the use of medication for behavioral expressions becomes the rare exception, rather than the rule.

The poet Maya Angelou said: "You did then what you knew how to do and when you knew better you did better" (Lowe, 1998, p. 132).

This book is for Simone.

Introduction

What It Isn't, What It Is

THIS BOOK IS NOT A PRIMER on dementia. It does not describe in detail the natural history of dementia, its symptoms, varieties, diagnosis, or treatment options. There are many authors who have done a thorough job of explaining these.

This is also not a review of the newest research studies attempting to find a cure or a means of arresting the progress of dementia. Like everyone, I hope we will find a cure for this devastating disease. Based on our history with other neurological diseases, however, we must accept the fact that such a cure may be slow in coming, and that there are millions of people living with dementia today who still need our care and attention.

If you have picked up this book, you may be a health care professional or a family member who cares for someone with dementia, or possibly you yourself have been diagnosed with some form of the disorder. You may have read other books about it, studied it for your career, listened to talk shows on dementia, or contacted your local Alzheimer's Association for more information. Perhaps you work in a care setting where dementia is prevalent.

My own work in elder care has followed a unique, dual pathway. As a board-certified internist and geriatrician and a full-time nursing home practitioner for over 18 years, I have treated thousands of people with all forms of dementia.

I am also an Educator for the Eden Alternative, the largest of the growing number of movements worldwide that are working to transform elder care, and with it our societal view of aging. Being both a practicing physician and an advocate of "culture change" in elder care puts me in a unique position to assemble all I have learned about the biomedical approach to dementia and reframe it within a new model of care.

Much of the information in this book comes from the pioneering efforts of other people whose work has greatly affected me. These people are too numerous to mention here, though you will read about them throughout the book. There are, however, a few individuals who have profoundly influenced my thinking.

Dr. William H. Thomas, a Harvard-trained physician, decided to try his hand at working in a nursing home in the early 1990s and became the architect of the Eden Alternative, which now boasts hundreds of member nursing homes in North America, Europe, Oceania, and Asia. Over 20,000 people have had formal training in the Eden philosophy and process and (along with other innovators, represented by organizations such as the Pioneer Network) they are turning our sterile institutions into vibrant, life-affirming homes where the frailest elders and their care partners can thrive and grow. Bill and his wife, Jude Meyers-Thomas, continue to be outspoken advocates for elders worldwide.

But the work of such pioneers represents only a few waves in an ocean of elder care settings around the world, and nowhere is the need for transformation more critical than in our care of people with dementia.

Another pioneer who deserves significant credit for my personal journey is the late Tom Kitwood, a psychologist who founded the Bradford Dementia Group in England, and whose "person-centered" approach to people with dementia has helped form much of the foundation for my further work. His group continues to serve as an important resource for a more humane, relationship-rich approach to people with dementia.

We need to do more than simply adjust our thinking about this disorder. We need to radically alter the way we look at the challenging behavioral expressions so commonly seen in people with dementia. As I will relate, our biomedical approach is inadequate to the needs of our rapidly increasing population living with dementia, and it compromises the well-being and personhood of millions of people around the world. It is only through a radical transformation of our system and approach to care that we can hope to turn the tide.

Thus I am adding yet another volume to the mountain of books on this common, life-altering condition. My hope is that this book will help rebalance our approach to people with dementia and motivate us to promote a change of direction in their care. The first part, Paradigms and Problems, looks at the current view of dementia and its behavioral expressions and reviews some alarming medication trends worldwide. Next, it examines the research upon which current prescribing patterns are based, but with a different perspective than most of the medical establishment has entertained thus far.

The next chapters in Part 1 describe in detail the problems with our current model of elder care. There are other books on culture change that address the topic very well, but I believe it is important to review this in a manner that speaks directly to the care of people with dementia.

There are those who believe that this topic doesn't require a lot of explanation because the problems with our institutional model of care are well known by now. I disagree. There are many people giving lip service to "culture change." Even the Centers for Medicare and Medicaid Services (CMS) has adopted the buzzword. But when it comes to the care of people with dementia, either our understanding of this concept is so limited or else our traditional approach is so deeply ingrained that we don't even realize how institutionalized our attitudes have become. In his video *Everyday Creativity* (1999), photographer Dewitt Jones observes that patterns and structures are "incredibly important. We can't function without them. But we all know that if we let these patterns go too long unquestioned, they become our prisons." For this reason, I will expend some effort to show that our approach to care needs a radical overhaul.

In the second part of the book, Shifts, we will use what we have learned to craft a new *experiential* model for viewing dementia. This model will enable us to create a world in which even people with advanced dementia can experience well-being and growth, with little or no medication. The chapters in this part will also begin to lay out the process for transforming from a biomedical to an experiential approach to care in all settings.

The final part, Solutions, applies the experiential model to offer some specific approaches to caring for people with dementia, and gives concrete suggestions for understanding and responding to many behavioral expressions that are commonly seen. The book closes with stories of people who are already making this transformation, whose successes will show us where we need to go.

I have an important reason for saving this discussion for the very end. Despite much information on nonpharmacological treatment of dementia, in practice most people fall back on medication use at some point. My work with the Eden Alternative has helped me to understand why this happens. Nonpharmacological approaches will never fully succeed until the underlying culture of care can be transformed. I cannot emphasize this enough. If you try to use the suggestions offered in the back of the book without doing any of the difficult and challenging work of truly changing the care environment, then you will not realize the full benefits. There are no gimmicks; this is not a "10 Quick Steps to Success" book. Hard work and dedication are required, but the need is critical and the rewards are great.

In my own practice, I have been able to care for people with dementia with only a small fraction of the psychiatric medication that most people use, even though St. John's Home is still at a fairly early stage in the transformational process. Sustaining such success, however, requires the ongoing effort of the entire organization.

Nevertheless, we can take these successes and the very real benefits that many of us have seen, and create a road map that shows where this journey can take us, if we dare to embark. This book will also explain what each of us can do today, no matter where we are, to take the first steps.

As I write these words, my wife and I—now "empty-nesters"—are in the process of downsizing to a smaller home. I have packed old files, mementos, and other pieces of "my life so far" into boxes. At some point after we relocate, I will simply unpack the boxes and retrieve the contents. But how would I feel if I opened a box and didn't find what I was looking for? What if one or more boxes were lost by the movers and I could never retrieve that piece of my life and all of its meaning?

This must be the dilemma of a person who faces progressive memory loss—the inability to retrieve important pieces of one's life, which can lead to a loss of self. After living with dementia for six years, Dr. Richard Taylor (2007) shared his experience:

> Sometimes, when I am alone with my thoughts, I wander aimlessly around the corridors of my mind. I open various doors to see if they

are still full of the memories I stored there years ago. To my pleasant surprise, most of them seem to contain all that I remember putting in the room. However, as I move from the past toward the present, I find more and more empty rooms. Not only are they empty, they are dark. They offer no clue, other than the label on the door, as to what they once contained.

 . . . It is very unnerving to be in the midst of a conversation and all of a sudden need to open the door to a room to access its contents and—the room is dark. I don't have a clue. (p. 35)

This loss of stored memories can be accompanied by the inability to perform other previously simple functions, such as balancing a checkbook, driving to the store, even putting on one's clothes in the morning. As I reflect on this, it is all too clear to me that if we are to provide the best care for people with dementia, we need to spend a lot more time trying to understand what it feels like to live with dementia. This is what I call an *experiential* approach to dementia, and it will challenge many of the "truths" that are shared about the disorder.

Warm-Up Exercise—"The Birthday Cake"

Before you shift paradigms, you may find it helpful to stretch your mind with a warm-up exercise. You have a problem. It's your birthday, and you are celebrating with seven of your close friends, one of whom has made a delicious chocolate cake. The baker, however, is a bit of a prankster. She has told you that you have to cut the cake in a special manner or else you can't have any. Your task is to cut the cake in eight pieces of equal size and shape, but you can only make three slices through the cake with your knife.

 Now, cutting a cake in eight pieces is not particularly difficult. Most of us do it the same way. Assuming the cake is round, you begin by cutting the cake at ninety-degree angles to split it into quarters:

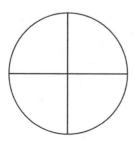

Next, you make two cuts on the diagonal, to split each of these pieces, creating eight equal wedges:

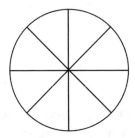

That's easy enough; the problem is that it took *four* cuts of the knife. How can you possibly do it with only three?

I've posed this problem in many teaching sessions, and it's a rare person who can get the answer quickly. After each group struggles for a while, I remind them that the drawings I have shown do not truly represent the cake, which of course is a three-dimensional object. Usually at this point, a couple of people will figure it out.

The answer, you see, is to start by cutting the cake in quarters with two slices of the knife as we did in the first figure above. The third slice, however, is cut through the side of the cake, as if making a horizontal cut between the layers of a two-layer cake. Now you have created eight pieces of equal size and shape, with only three cuts of the knife.

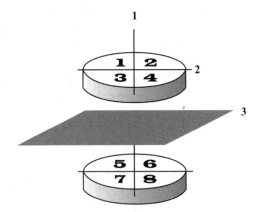

Why is this so hard to grasp at the outset? The reason, of course, is that no one ever cuts a cake this way. We have a system for cutting a cake into slices. Each of us has our own style, but we all tend to look down at the cake from above. In doing so, we view the top of the cake as a two-dimensional surface and plan our cuts from this point of view. That works fine until someone asks us to "think outside the box." Then, our habits blind us to other possibilities.

So why did I start a book on dementia with a puzzle about cutting birthday cake? Dementia is becoming increasingly common as our population ages; it will affect tens of millions of people worldwide over the next few decades. Our approach to this problem, however, has been to design a badly flawed system of care that isolates elders with dementia at home or moves them into cold institutional settings. Both situations fail to create the environment a person needs in order to thrive, and our response to their distress is to overmedicate and sedate them. The more that people with dementia suffer, the more we pile on the medications and institutionalize their lives.

Like the birthday cake, we look at the person with dementia from a single viewpoint—that of a broken person in need of medication to mitigate the decline. Our standardized tests reduce the personhood of the elder to a list of disordered thinking processes, while we ignore the complex cognitive and emotional qualities that can be retained even in advanced stages of the disorder. As a result, our attempts to treat dementia involve repeating or intensifying failed strategies, and like the person who keeps trying to cut the cake from the top, we never succeed in finding a solution.

Part of the disability of dementia lies in the disorder itself, which robs people of the capacity to experience and enjoy life as they have in the past. However, another disability of the disorder is the way our medical and social systems further deprive each person of the chance to truly grow and thrive despite his or her limitations.

Much attention is paid to the frosting and decorations that adorn a birthday cake. Yet only when we cut into the cake do we discover the rich substance that lies beneath the surface. In this book you will discover novel ways to "cut the cake" to discover the rich tapestry that exists within each individual.

By creating a world that provides more holistic care and nurtures individual growth, we can reclaim lives and restore hope—not only for those who live with dementia, but also for their families and other care partners. Do you care for one or more people with dementia? Do you feel frustrated by the suffering that persists despite the best medical treatments? Then make a wish. Blow out the candles. And read on. . . .

PART 1

Paradigms
and Problems

CHAPTER 1

The Universe
of Dementia

And What Lies Beyond

The only true voyage of discovery . . . would be not to visit
strange lands, but to possess other eyes, to behold the universe through the eyes of another, of a hundred others, to
behold the hundred universes that each of them beholds,
that each of them is.

(Marcel Proust, The Captive)

THE WORLD'S POPULATION is aging. Between the years 2000 and 2030,
the number of Americans over age 65 will double. The same is true for
Americans over age 85 (Administration on Aging, 2008). In recently
emerging economies such as Singapore, those numbers will increase by
more than *fivefold* in the same time period.

As the number of older people increases, the numbers of people
with Alzheimer's disease and other forms of dementia will follow suit.
Although estimates vary for these earliest years of the 21st century, it is
safe to say that over 5 million Americans currently live with some form
of dementia. This number will grow more than threefold by 2050 to
about 16 million. Worldwide, as many as 100 million people may have
dementia by that time (Alzheimer's Disease International, 2009).

These numbers will change, of course, if an effective prevention or
cure is found. So far, however, most treatments have centered on trying
to mitigate the decline of people who already have the disease. Based
on the multiplicity of risk factors, the many forms of dementia, and our
history with most degenerative diseases, an out-and-out cure seems

unlikely anytime soon. I don't say this to be overly pessimistic, or to discourage further research in these areas. I say this to acknowledge the reality that dementia is likely to be around on a large scale for a long time. This book is in part a call to action to devote much more time and effort to improving the lives of millions of people who are living with dementia today or who will develop the condition in years to come.

There are few, if any, illnesses regarded with as much dread as Alzheimer's disease. It is not uncommon for people to say that they would rather die from a rapidly fatal disease than live for many years with dementia. If you browse the issues of most popular magazines, you can find articles telling you how you can continue to live a rich and fulfilling life in spite of a diagnosis of cancer, diabetes, paraplegia, or almost any other incurable condition. You never see such articles about Alzheimer's. Why is that? Our dread of Alzheimer's arises in part from the nature of the disease itself, with the feared losses of memory and meaningful connections, even of a lost sense of self that can occur. But our dread also reflects the kind of life that our care system has created for people who receive the diagnosis. This is the hidden tragedy of dementia, and one that we must work hard to reverse.

In their book *The Myth of Alzheimer's* (2008), authors Dr. Peter Whitehouse and Daniel George question the way this condition has been categorized. They even question whether Alzheimer's is a disease, or is instead a part of the overall spectrum of brain aging. Theirs is a fascinating book, but I am going to resist the urge to ask this same question in mine. Regardless of how we choose to classify the various forms of dementia, I agree wholeheartedly that the narrow biomedical view has created a system of care that produces as much disability as the disorder itself.

Dementia is more than neuropathology. Of course, you can examine the brain of a person with Alzheimer's and see characteristic protein plaques and tangled nerve cells. But just as there is a difference between *brain* and *mind*, there is also a difference between *brain disease* and *the experience of dementia*.

Musician and cognitive psychologist Daniel Levitin (2006) distinguishes *mind* and *brain* in this manner:

> For cognitive scientists, the word *mind* refers to that part of each of us that embodies our thoughts, hopes, desires, memories, beliefs and experiences. The brain, on the other hand, is an organ of the body, a

collection of cells and water, chemicals and blood vessels that resides in the skull. Activity in the brain gives rise to the contents of the mind. . . . [D]ifferent minds can arise from very similar brains. (p. 81)

With our biomedical approach, we tend to characterize dementia as a list of impairments in brain function, such as memory, orientation, calculation, shape recognition, word finding, or sentence formation. In doing so, we reduce the person to a series of discrete cognitive tasks that can or cannot be performed. We forget that dementia has other components—existential, spiritual, and experiential. In fact, it is hard to discuss one of these facets without bringing the others into play.

The popular on-line reference Wikipedia defines an *existential crisis* (2009) as "a perceived sense of harsh confrontation experienced when a human confronts questions of existence and a change in one's subjective perception (of) their relation to their world." It sounds like a description of the experience of a person who has been diagnosed with dementia. Among the listed causes of such a crisis are "the sense of being alone and isolated in the world, a new-found grasp or appreciation of one's mortality, and believing that one's life has no purpose or external meaning." An existential crisis may therefore describe how the *mind* reacts to the changes caused by dementia in the *brain*. It also reflects how people react to changes in the way they are viewed by those around them. This, then, is the "experiential universe" that stretches far beyond the physical changes of dementia. Our biomedical view does not have a powerful enough lens to see this part of the universe.

Moreover, as the opening quote by Proust implies, there are many universes to consider, because seeing dementia from the standpoint of experience requires taking each individual's life history into account, and it creates a unique path for each individual, regardless of the common diagnosis.

When Dr. William Thomas conceived of the Eden Alternative approach to transforming nursing homes, he started with an important realization: In spite of our advances in geriatric medicine, advanced training in many disciplines, and multiple levels of regulation and oversight, people in nursing homes still suffer on a daily basis. The reason for this is that nursing homes operate in a limited universe—one that sees and treats medical illness. Thomas saw that people also struggle with diseases of the human *spirit*. He identified three plagues of institutionalized adults: loneliness, helplessness, and boredom. Everyone experiences these conditions from time to time, but institutionalized people are at a much higher risk, and they have fewer resources with which to combat them. In fact, the institutional approach to care is not only inadequate to address these plagues, but also actually contributes to them.

The Eden Alternative (along with other philosophies of culture change in nursing homes) believes that people suffer more on a day-to-day basis from these conditions than from their medical illnesses. Accordingly, if we create a care environment that addresses these plagues, we can create a more enjoyable, meaningful life, even if we cannot cure the medical illnesses.

As an Eden Alternative Educator, I will use these ideas as my jumping-off point for expanding the view of dementia. I will follow a parallel line of reasoning: that our approach to dementia only sees medical symptoms that require medical treatments, that our medical approach actually *increases* individuals' suffering, and that a new approach can create a life worth living, even as dementia progresses to later stages.

This is a far cry from the current view of dementia. To illustrate this further, let's try a brief exercise.

Diabetes versus Dementia

Imagine for a few moments that you have been diagnosed with diabetes. I am choosing this disease because it is a common condition about which most of us have a fair degree of awareness. It is incurable, but treatments are available. Many people live many years without serious problems, but many people may experience progression of the disease or develop serious complications.

Imagine that you are not feeling quite right, and so you visit your physician to find out what is wrong. After an examination and some testing, the doctor discovers that it is likely that diabetes is the culprit. Of course, any new diagnosis can lead to emotional upset. There is a realization that your body is changing, that you are no longer free of illness, that you may need medication and will need to change your lifestyle. The disease could affect your life and longevity in many ways.

Now let's add another wrinkle to the scenario. How would you feel if your doctor insisted that your spouse, son, or daughter accompany you to your follow-up visit? The doctor speaks to your family member instead of directly to you, and says:

Your loved one has diabetes. This is an incurable and progressive disease that can produce complications and may well lead to your loved one's death. I think that you need to start thinking about planning for when your loved one can no longer do things alone, and start talking about advanced directives for end-of-life care.

I doubt that most people receive the news of diabetes in such dire terms. And yet this is common when someone receives a diagnosis of dementia, even when it is in its very early stages.

Next, imagine that as a result of this single doctor visit people start treating you differently and include you less in activities and family decisions, even though you want to participate. "The loneliest thing in the world is to be standing when everyone around you is sitting . . . and they all look at you and ask, 'What is wrong with her?'" These are the words of Diana Friel McGowin, who documented her own experience with the diagnosis of Alzheimer's disease in her book *Living in the Labyrinth* (1993, p. 80).

Finally, imagine that from this day on, everything you do, from driving your car to paying your bills, is being scrutinized closely, and if there is the slightest slip—the fender bender we have all had to deal with, the occasional late bill payment, the inability to name a familiar song—you are in danger of having your independence taken from you.

It is hard to imagine these things happening to a diabetic. They happen every day to someone with a new diagnosis of dementia.

I am not suggesting that a person who can't remember her children's names should be out driving a car. But dementia is a powerful label that starts a long slide into a world of disempowerment, often long before abilities are lost. McGowin continues, "My diagnosis exposed me to the elements. My rights had become tenuous and delicate. They existed only so long as nothing untoward occurred" (pp. 82–83).

Indeed, our prevailing view of dementia is that it is tragic, costly, and burdensome. Even as Alzheimer's advocates campaign for more funding and resources, there is a tendency to express the urgency of the need by emphasizing the tragedy of dementia. I have heard the very people who are charged with helping those with dementia to live better lives describe the disease as a "living death" or "the worst illness a person can have." Unfortunately, this approach only creates additional barriers.

The dementia-as-tragedy dialogue increases public fear of the disorder, which is a barrier to education. It also heightens the stigma of the disease, which is a barrier to early detection. ~~After all, who would want to be diagnosed, knowing they will be treated like less of a person when the results are in?~~ For doctors and other care professionals, this view of dementia causes us to see people primarily for their illness, rather than as unique individuals who happen to share a diagnosis. For researchers and the entities that fund them, it puts most resources into seeking the "Holy Grails" of prevention and cure, while comparatively little is given to help improve the lives of those millions of people who live with dementia that will neither be prevented nor cured.

To paraphrase Dr. William Thomas's frequent comment about aging, "It is time for a new dialogue" on dementia. Accordingly, this book will bring the philosophies of the culture change movement to bear on our approach to dementia. It will also focus on the many expressions of the dementia experience that are commonly viewed as behavioral problems and try to see them with "other eyes." You will thereby hopefully come to see that these expressions reflect more than imbalances of brain chemicals and why, therefore, our medication approach does so little to create true well-being. In the larger universe of experience lie the true solutions.

A Few Words About Culture Change and Dementia

I want to answer a question that is no doubt on the minds of many readers: Why devote so much space to culture change principles in a book about dementia?

I have mentioned that, in spite of my disenchantment with medical treatment of behavioral expressions, the nonpharmacological alternatives often fall short in practice. That is because these interventions are brief and do not change the underlying environment experienced by the person with dementia throughout every day and night of life. ~~For example, validation techniques are often taught as an approach to repetitive requests, such as wanting to go home or asking for a loved one.~~ As St. John's Home has transformed away from the traditional medical model, ~~we have seen how our move to permanent staffing (in order to develop close, continuing relationships) has enhanced the power of such interventions to take hold. A stranger who tries to validate your distress won't hold as much weight as a friend.~~

~~I hope to make clear the necessity to *transform* the institutional model in order to maximize your success at caring for people with dementia. I'll repeat myself—transformation is the foundation of~~

enlightened care. The institutional model will *never* succeed in this endeavor. What we need is not a faster caterpillar; we need a butterfly.

Furthermore, you will come to see that the word *institution* means much more than a building. This book will show how care in one's own home can be just as institutional as in a nursing home.

The term *culture change* is often misunderstood. Unfortunately, the words *culture* and *change* can be problematic. They are often understood to mean changing personal culture—family values and religious beliefs. It is important to emphasize that this is not the case.

Organizations also have a culture—a predominating system of attitudes, values, and beliefs that inform daily operations (Fox, 2007). We must be careful to emphasize that the system is broken, not the people.

Much of what is written about the culture change movement can sound like nursing home bashing, so it is worth reminding people that I also work in a nursing home—one that still retains many institutional trappings. There is no place where more caring, compassionate people can be found than in the field of elder care. It is important to emphasize this point, because this is a challenging book. It is common for people to feel offended by statements that our approach needs to change; they often feel like they are being told they have not been providing high-quality, compassionate care.

In discussing how a care approach can be transformed, I find it helpful to share with people the example of how the medical treatment of stomach ulcers has changed. In the 1950s, a person with an ulcer was likely told to drink milk and Maalox and to eat soda crackers. Several operations were devised to cut out stomach ulcers or to cut the nerves that increase stomach acid secretion. In the 1970s, "H_2 blocker" drugs were developed, starting with cimetidine. Many other similar drugs followed. The result was a sudden drop in the need for ulcer surgery. Eventually, proton pump inhibitor drugs such as omeprazole improved results even further. In the 1980s, an Australian named Barry Marshall got the crazy notion that ulcers might be caused by an infection. He had seen bacteria in the stomachs of many people with ulcers (it is not normal for bacteria to live in the stomach), but he could not find a suitable way to devise a cause-and-effect study. He began drinking solutions containing the bacteria and was ultimately able to document the onset of indigestion and the development of erosions in his own stomach, which he later cured with antibiotics. Now we treat most ulcers with antibiotics. (Marshall won the Nobel Prize in medicine in 2005.)

This story demonstrates that a knowledge base changes with time. Doctors in the 1950s were neither stupid nor uncaring. As new information emerges, a care and treatment approach changes as well. Similarly, culture change gives us a new paradigm for improving elder care in the future; and with this comes a new paradigm for approaching the care of people who live with dementia.

I tell care staff that they are like fine musicians who are being forced to play their instruments while wearing gloves. They may hit a few beautiful notes, but much of the time, in spite of all of their effort and care, they know they are not quite creating the music they want to hear. If we wish to truly spark a lasting change and free ourselves of our constraints, sometimes it is necessary to "drop the gloves."

So while I continue to care deeply for my colleagues in medicine and elder care, this book will frankly point out the shortcomings of the approaches we have all been taught over the years. As in the Angelou quote in the Prologue, we must do better.

Change is also frightening for many people. Truthfully, change can be either good or bad, and the word itself should not necessarily conjure up positive or negative images. In 1963, Bob Dylan wrote "The Times They Are a-Changin'," presaging a tumultuous period in our nation's history. But was the song predicting positive or negative changes? The answer depends, in part, on whom you ask. The lyrics to Dylan's song certainly succeeded in communicating the passion and urgency of his message. But the words were also full of strife—images of battles, generational misunderstandings, and changes in our nation's power structure. It could be a stirring song for one listener and terrifying for another. Perhaps it was a little of both.

This illustrates why change often creates a less-than-enthusiastic response. People fear change for many reasons. The greatest reason is the loss of control that may accompany the change (is change being done *by* me, or *to* me?). There is a great deal of fear of the unknown. People are reluctant to disrupt their patterns and routines. Once again, this is not because of any failing on our part. Resistance to change is hardwired into our DNA. Our ability to resist severe changes in our body temperature, fluid balance, and electrolyte levels is essential to human survival. These survival mechanisms carry over to our patterns of behavior. People put a lot of stock in maintaining a comfort zone— so much so that they will often accept a bad situation rather than take a chance on changing to a better one. After all, it could be worse!

Regarding our fear of change, Dr. William Thomas (2008) once remarked, "Sometimes we build 'comfortable prisons' for ourselves."

I find that a better word than *change* for what we wish to accomplish is *growth*. Growth is more holistic and almost always carries positive connotations. Growth can certainly be painful at times and it doesn't always proceed smoothly, but we usually see it as a path to a better outcome. We want to grow and to encourage growth in others. We may fear change, but we must acknowledge that growth requires change. You can change without growing, but you cannot grow without changing. When we refuse to change, we cease to grow.

The antidote to fear is education. The key is to help each person to understand the change, and then to manage it by creating a pathway that allows every care partner to give input into the process, and, finally, to monitor their progress on the journey.

I wrote this book to empower everyone whose life or career has been touched by dementia to grow as partners in creating a better life for all involved.

CHAPTER 2

The Pill Paradigm

A Critical Look at Medication Use

THIS IMPORTANT CHAPTER reviews the major research upon which our drug prescribing patterns are based. These studies have led to the use of psychiatric medication for millions of people with dementia. Unfortunately, they have led us to adopt a care approach that is seriously flawed and that usually produces more harm than good.

Much of the discussion addresses the use of antipsychotic drugs, as these are the most commonly used and carry the most risks. Most of my arguments regarding the use of these medications can be applied to the other types of psychiatric drugs as well.

I have intentionally avoided the use of medical jargon in this chapter in order to present a viewpoint that will be clear to every reader, regardless of medical background. Even if you have no medical background, please try to read through this discussion, with the understanding that transforming an approach to care is hard work, and it will not happen unless you are convinced that the medication approach is neither safe nor effective. The chapter concludes with some of the most remarkable stories from my clinical experience.

Antipsychotic Drugs

Background

Schizophrenia is a serious, disabling disorder that affects more than 2 million Americans. The development and refinement of antipsychotic medications have literally been lifesaving for many people who live with this disease. Antipsychotic drugs have been used for dementia because many people develop abnormal thought processes at some point, including some that resemble the paranoia, delusions, and hallucinations of schizophrenics. But the majority of people with dementia are medicated with antipsychotic drugs for other behavioral symptoms, including agitation, aggression, anxiety, pacing, and repetitive speech.

The Omnibus Budget and Reconciliation Act of 1987 contained specific language addressing the rising concern that these and other psychotropic drugs were being overused in nursing homes. This law challenges care professionals to be sure that all such drugs are used only to treat specific medical symptoms and not as a matter of staff convenience or as a substitute for care. After this law was enacted, the prevalence of antipsychotic drug use dropped by an average of 30% across nursing homes in the United States (Snowden and Roy-Byrne, 1998). By 1995, only 16% of people in nursing homes were prescribed antipsychotic medication (Briesacher et al., 2005). However, the 1990s also saw the release of a new generation of atypical antipsychotic drugs. These drugs were developed to reduce some of the major side effects seen with the older drugs, such as muscle rigidity and dyskinesias (uncontrollable movements).

The first atypical drug, clozapine, was released in the United States in 1989 but saw very limited use in dementia care due to its potential for toxic effects on the bone marrow. Risperidone was released in 1993, and six similar drugs have been approved since. Because these drugs were purported to be safer alternatives to the older drugs, their use in dementia care skyrocketed over the next 2 decades, and the prevalence of antipsychotic drug use in nursing homes began to reverse its previous downward trend. A study of the 2.4 million Medicare recipients who spent any time in a nursing home from 2000 to 2001 showed that 28% (or 693,000 people) were prescribed an antipsychotic medication, nearly doubling the number from 5 years previous (Briesacher et al., 2005). Furthermore, fewer than half of those people were given the medications in accordance with national nursing home prescribing guidelines, and nearly a quarter had *no* appropriate indication for the pill. Most disturbing was the finding that 17.2% (over 100,000 frail older adults) received more than the maximum recommended daily dose. Similar statistics are not available for more recent years, but a look at our prescribing trends suggests that this number has continued to rise significantly. There continues to be a rapid rise in the use of these medications across the United States in spite of fairly stable numbers of people with other kinds of psychiatric disorders.

Sales of antipsychotic drugs doubled from $5.3 billion to $10.4 billion between 2001 and 2005, costing Medicaid more dollars than were spent on heart medications or antibiotics (Briesacher et al., 2005). The actual number of prescriptions written each year increased from 29.9 million to 43.8 million in the same interval (IMS Health, 2006). That's a ratio of about 20 prescriptions written for every person with schizophrenia in the United States!

So who is getting all of these extra prescriptions? Some are given to people with serious episodes of depression. Some are used for the manic symptoms that can accompany bipolar disease. Some are used for the delirium that can accompany acute illnesses or can occur during a terminal illness. But many, if not most, are given to treat the "challenging behaviors" of dementia. In fact, this is the only group of people whose increase in numbers over time has mirrored the rapid increase in antipsychotic drug prescriptions. (It is impossible to track the exact number used for this purpose, as these drugs are not approved by the U.S. Food and Drug Administration for use in dementia care.)

This pattern of use is reflected globally as well. According to the Danish Medicines Agency, 28% of people in Danish nursing homes (with and without dementia) were on antipsychotics in 2003 (Danish Medicines Agency, 2005). In Sydney, Australia, that same year, over 25% of the residents of their 40 nursing homes were treated with antipsychotics, and 80% of those treated did not have a diagnosis of psychosis (Snowden, Day, and Baker, 2005). A Canadian study of nearly 20,000 adults over age 65 admitted to nursing homes (with no prior history of psychosis or antipsychotic drug use) showed that 17% were put on an antipsychotic drug within the first 100 days and 24% within a year (Bronskill et al., 2004). A 2005 report showed a nearly 35% increase in antipsychotic prescriptions for older adults in Ontario, Canada, from 1993 to 2002, associated with a cost increase of 749% (Rapoport, Mamdani, Shulman, Herrmann, and Rochon, 2005). If we look only at people with a diagnosis of dementia living in nursing homes in the industrialized nations of the world, we find that similar proportions—about 40%—are receiving antipsychotic drugs (Margallo-Lana et al., 2001).

The pharmaceutical industry is clearly positioned for a drastic increase in the use of these newer antipsychotic drugs. A May 2006 *Psychiatric News* Web post indicated that there are as many as 40 new agents in the research and development pipeline (*Psychiatric News*, 2006). Since the number of people with psychiatric illness is rising much more slowly than our population with dementia, one could conclude that the drug industry believes this to be the future of dementia treatment.

Given the magnitude of the use of antipsychotic drugs to treat dementia, it must be determined that these medications produce a benefit of similar magnitude to justify the huge cost and potential side effects. I will start with a general review of the medication trials to date. Then I will discuss several factors that challenge many of the benefits claimed.

Studies of Antipsychotic Drugs in Dementia Care

It is worth mentioning at the outset that virtually all of the studies that claim to show a benefit of antipsychotic drugs in dementia care have been sponsored by the companies that manufactured the study drugs. This is more often the case with modern drug trials, and this fact does not in and of itself invalidate the results. However, recent independent studies suggest that these claims require a more critical look.

An extensive paper in the *Journal of the American Medical Association* reviewed the best-designed studies of drug therapy for behavioral symptoms of dementia that had been published over the previous 40 years (Sink, Holden, and Yaffe, 2005). The conclusion for all types of drugs was that there was very limited benefit, if any, and that our medication approach was "not particularly effective" (p. 596).

A study of community-dwelling adults with dementia in the *New England Journal of Medicine* concluded that, in the case of antipsychotic drugs, the risks outweighed the benefits for behavioral symptoms of dementia, including people with delusional symptoms and aggression (Schneider et al., 2006). An accompanying editorial softened the conclusion a bit by suggesting that there may still be subgroups of people that will benefit, but that such treatment was best provided in settings "that can provide the skill and expertise needed to ensure that the *risks associated with the drugs are justified by their potential benefits*" (Karlawish,

2006, p. 1605). (The emphasis is mine—I think it is significant that *risks* was placed before *potential benefits* in that phrase.) Not a particularly ringing endorsement.

Among the risks of antipsychotic drugs are the well-known problems with movement disorders and gait imbalance. (These side effects still exist in the newer drugs, although to a lesser extent.) All antipsychotic drugs produce a fair amount of sedation as well, which in turn can cause a host of adverse effects, including inadequate food and fluid intake, falls and fractures, incontinence, infections, and bedsores. But it doesn't end there. More recent studies have suggested increased risks of stroke (Gill et al., 2005; Wooltorton, 2002; Wooltorton, 2004); increased risk of pneumonia (Knol et al., 2008); faster cognitive decline (Ballard et al., 2005; McShane et al., 1997); and even an increased rate of death, independent of the underlying disease process (Gill et al., 2007; Kales et al., 2007; Schneider, Dagerman, and Insel, 2005). Most recently, a U.K. study showed that, over a 3-year period, people with dementia who were given antipsychotic drugs had *double* the mortality of those who were given a placebo (Ballard et al., 2009).

Antipsychotic drugs would have to work very well to justify so much risk. Unfortunately, they don't.

Do Antipsychotics Work?

This section examines the published studies in more detail and, in keeping with the theme of this book, considers some alternate ways of interpreting the data—an approach to analysis that is rarely if ever found in medical journals. The placebo effect is remarkable in these studies, and there are also some important aspects of study design, measurement, and conclusions that warrant discussion.

High Placebo Responses

To publish a well-regarded drug intervention study, it is best to compare the results to a group of people taking a placebo drug and to "blind" the observers such that they do not know which pill each person is receiving. If an observer knows that a person is taking the actual drug, there might be a tendency to report a better outcome than for those on the placebo. By blinding the study, this bias is eliminated. In addition, the people taking the pills might be more inclined to report positive effects if they know that they are taking the actual drug. Therefore, the participants are also blinded as to which pills they are taking.

The other reason for using a placebo group is that good or bad symptoms might occur due to random factors not related to the drug. Such symptoms would be expected to happen as often with both the study drug group and the placebo group. For example, if 10% of the people taking a study drug develop nausea and vomiting, it could be an important side effect of the drug. But if 10% of the people on the placebo also vomit, then it is more likely that it was due to another cause, such as a gastrointestinal virus running through the community.

Traditionally, reported improvements in most placebo groups can start as high as 30%. Then they tend to decrease over time. Many people may feel better on a pill due to the hope that they are on the study drug. Over time, however, this desire for improvement may be overshadowed by the reality that the pill hasn't truly helped their symptoms.

One striking feature of the studies most often quoted to support antipsychotic drug use is that all of the placebo responses are very high, nearly as high as the study drug results. These responses usually run in the range of 30% to 40%, but sometimes reach 50% or higher. This is a figure that demands investigation and yet has received little attention.

Keep in mind that most people studied for behavioral symptoms of dementia have fairly advanced disease. Most of these people were enrolled by proxy and did not understand the study protocol—indeed, most probably didn't even know they were in a study or taking a new medication. It follows that such people would not have the expectation of improvement that characterizes much of the usual placebo effect. One would therefore conclude that the response to a placebo in these studies should be lower than that in other drug studies in which sub-jects are well aware of the study design. Instead, we see the opposite. In fact, the placebo response in these studies either stays level or even increases over time—in one study it reached a final level of 61% (De Deyn et al., 1999). What is it about people with dementia that makes them different?

I think there are two factors at work here. First, there is increased attention paid to people in studies, with regular visits for observation and assessment. This added attention may fulfill some of the need for human interaction that is so often lacking for those with dementia in institutional environments. Second, drug studies usually take weeks or months to complete. In that time period, many people with dementia have had time to adjust to their new environment and create more last-ing familiarity with the staff and with the layout of the facility.

Cohen-Mansfield and Mintzer (2005) contrast the proponents of a biochemical theory of behavioral symptoms with those who feel that the care environment is the prime determinant. They conclude that the presence of the "strong placebo response" shows that these are not mutually exclusive concepts. In other words, it follows that the care environment can produce striking neurochemical changes.

Why is this so important? Because these studies have consistently shown that 30% to 60% of people with behavioral symptoms get better simply from the passage of time, and from the increased attention of their care partners. No other features of enlightened care were added to these studies. Imagine the additional improvement we might see if we were to radically improve the care environment for people with dementia!

> Specifically, evidence shows that a large proportion of these so-called behavior problems stem from an incongruence between the needs of the people who suffer from dementia and the degree to which their environment fulfills those needs. Thus many "problematic behaviors" represent a cry for help, a result of unmet needs, or an inadequate attempt to fulfill those needs (Cohen-Mansfield and Mintzer, 2005, p. 37).

Does Anyone Benefit from Antipsychotic Drugs?

If you combine the results of the most-quoted drug trials for behavioral symptoms, you will find that the overall response rate is only about 18% higher than that for placebo (Karlawish, 2006). In other words, even if we take these studies at face value, fewer than one in five people will improve due to the medication. How many doctors would give a patient an antibiotic that has less than a 20% chance of working, or a heart medication that helps fewer than one in five patients?

Further examination of these drug studies reveals that even the 18% figure likely overestimates the number of people that truly benefit. There are several reasons for this. As previously mentioned, virtually all of these studies were supported by the manufacturers of the drug being tested. This is worth repeating because a multitude of decisions go into designing a study: what types of dementia and behavioral symptoms to address, whom to include and exclude, how to measure positive and negative effects, how to analyze the data, which results or end points to measure, and so forth. Each decision point creates an opportunity for investigational bias to occur.

There is also bias in the choice of which studies will be submitted or accepted for publication. A recent study of published antidepressant trials should give us pause. This study found that of 74 antidepressant trials reported to the Food and Drug Administration, only 51% had positive results, but 94% of those that were published in medical journals were either positive studies or else questionable studies that were reframed in a more positive light (Turner, Matthews, Linardatos, Tell, and Rosenthal, 2008). The study also suggests that even bias enters into the wording of results. Most published antipsychotic studies contain conclusions whose wording suggests that the study drug "is safe and effective for the treatment of behavioral symptoms of dementia," putting the results in a positive light. However, one could report these same results and state that the study drug "causes significant amounts of sedation and gait imbalance, and fewer than one in five people show any improvement." As you can see, how you report the results leaves a lot of room for interpretation. A busy physician reading either of those two conclusions could have very different thoughts about the usefulness of the drug.

Another problem with these studies is that few of the primary goals that were measured were actually achieved by the drugs. Many of the "improvements" reported were only found through secondary, or post hoc, analysis of the data, which was conducted when the drug failed to achieve the primary goal. Once again, this opens up the studies to criticism.

Two other factors, however, the negative end points and the sedation factor, raise the most serious concerns about the validity of these studies.

Negative End Points

Many rating scales are used to measure the behavioral expressions of dementia. Examples include the BEHAVE-AD (Reisberg et al., 1987) and the Cohen-Mansfield Agitation Inventory (Cohen-Mansfield, Marx, and Rosenthal, 1989). Each scale has its advantages and disadvantages, but all have one major drawback: They only measure the presence, absence, or degree of *negative* (undesirable) symptoms. As such, all drug intervention trials attempt to show a decrease in these negative symptoms.

Why is this critical? The first reason is that the studies do not measure positive outcomes, such as *well-being*, as a result of the medication. We would want to see a significant improvement in measures of well-being in order to justify the risks of the drugs, but one rarely sees this discussed.

The Sedation Question

There is another reason why it is not enough to measure only negative behavioral symptoms. If all we look for is a reduction in negative symptoms, then we can never completely rule out sedation as the reason for any "improvements" in behavior that we see. Do people who receive the drug feel a sense of ease in their environment? Do they show more signs of pleasure, feel more secure, show personal growth or heightened engagement with their surroundings? Or are they just quieter?

Studies of antipsychotic drugs tend to report significant amounts of sedation, usually ranging from 10% to nearly 30% of people on the medication. This raises two questions: Is that all? Does this account for the reported "improvement"? Only a few of the studies try to answer this question directly. Two of the most quoted drug trials state that the drugs' benefits remained positive even after removing the people who experienced sedation from the data analysis (De Deyn et al., 1999; Katz et al., 1999). But how did they decide who was overly sedated? Both studies measured it by self-report—this in populations whose average cognitive scores put them in the severe stage, where both language and comprehension can be compromised.

A broad spectrum exists between alertness and somnolence. If a person doesn't appear somnolent, it doesn't mean that she is not sedated. Anyone who has taken an antihistamine, a cold remedy, or a strong painkiller can tell you that, even though they may appear normal to their friends and coworkers, they often feel like they are "in a fog."

A review of medications for overactive bladder (Kay et al., 2005) reports that even in adults without dementia, these commonly used medications can cause significant cognitive impairment, along with electroencephalographic evidence of sedation. Furthermore, the authors state that such people are often unaware of these effects. Like antipsychotics, these bladder medications can block the brain transmitter acetylcholine, which is already reduced in people with dementia. (Older adults have only half the brain receptors for acetylcholine that younger adults have, and with dementia the amount is even less.)

Studies of commonly prescribed sleep aids (such as zolpidem and triazolam) in healthy adults without dementia showed that the subjects had lower performance on various cognitive tests than those who did not use them (Rush and Griffiths, 1996). Significant effects were seen even after a *single dose* of the medication (Mintzer, Frey, Yingling, and Griffiths, 1997; Mintzer and Griffiths, 1999; Otmani et al., 2008).

Thus the bottom line is that, unless we show an improvement in positive end points, we cannot rule out the effect of sedation.

Many who care for people with dementia will tell you that an antipsychotic medication may reduce episodes of agitation or aggression, but the result is rarely an alert, engaging, relaxed individual. As I related in my opening story of Simone, a lot of people on these medications give the observer a sense that "the light is on but nobody's home." Subtle changes in functional ability or language skills may be the only clues that the pill is causing sedation or worsening cognitive decline.

When they document the effects of these medications, observers often report that a person is "calm," but it is usually not the same as when you or I feel calm. I call it "calmatose." Consider this question: Who is in worse condition—the person who is expressing her needs by being vocal or lashing out during care, or the person who is always quiet, disengaged, and does not resist any care? According to Cohen-Mansfield and Mintzer (2005):

> [R]educing the behavior via sedation with psychoactive medication can be detrimental because it robs people with dementia of the very limited resources they have in either expressing or attending to their needs, and thereby diminishes the ability of caretakers to detect and address the true underlying need." (p. 38)

When considering the use of any psychotropic drug for a behavioral expression, it is important to ask how the drug is going to solve the problem. Is there something about the way the drug lowers dopamine levels in the brain that makes a wandering person stop wanting to explore his or her environment, or that makes a person who hates being bathed suddenly find the experience more enjoyable? This seems unlikely.

The challenge is to explain the mechanisms behind the drugs in use, particularly when a mismatch with the care environment is clearly triggering the distress. Other than in cases of true psychosis, it is difficult to reach any conclusion except that we are *sedating the behavior, and therefore the person.*

Consider the case of Ana A. Powers. As reported in *Democrat and Chronicle* on September 12, 2008 from Rochester, New York:

In court today, home-based day care operator Ana A. Powers was sentenced to two years in prison after being convicted of drugging the children in her charge. She was arrested in July 2007, after it was found that she had been giving the children strawberry-flavored milk laced with a sedating antihistamine to quiet them down. (Zeigler, 2008, pp. A1, A6)

Ms. Powers stated that "never in my mind or in my heart was [I] trying to hurt these children. I loved these children." Apparently, the children became "rowdy" in the afternoon, and she felt she needed to quiet them to allow her to get some of her work done. "I was just overwhelmed by the children and their issues," she added. The public was outraged and the assistant district attorney, calling Ms. Powers a monster, had requested the maximum punishment of 21 years in prison.

I don't consider Ms. Powers a monster. I think she was a woman who took on a task that she did not have the ability to handle, became overwhelmed, and made a very foolish choice, for which she is paying dearly. How can I feel so lenient? Because I see a similar drama played out every day, all across the country, by caring people. The only difference is that the drug recipients are people with dementia, not preschoolers. They live in nursing homes, assisted living apartments, and their own homes. And many of their caregivers are also overwhelmed by behavioral expressions they do not know how to handle, except by giving sedating medications. The only difference is that there is no public outrage.

Cause and Effect

Another pitfall in using medication for behavioral expressions is the risk of misinterpreting cause and effect. The varying rhythms of people with dementia require close observation in order to accurately decide what can or cannot be accomplished with medication use. I have seen several instances where the effects of treatment were misinterpreted.

To illustrate the confusion of cause and effect, let's consider the same person with dementia living in two different nursing homes. This gentleman will experience the same week in each home, and we will see the different ways in which each staff responds.

A Tale of Two Nursing Homes

In Nursing Home #1, the staff is observing Charlie for a week and not giving him any medication. On Sunday, Charlie has a bad day. He has little to stimulate him and his wife is unable to visit due to a stomach bug. He is restless and agitated. Efforts to redirect him do not allay his agitation, and he resists any attempts to have him sit still. The floating weekend nurses and aides are unfamiliar to him and don't know his wife is sick. He continues to pace throughout the evening and is up repeatedly at night, looking for his wife.

On Monday, Charlie continues to look a bit anxious, but the regular aides are back on duty, and he accepts some breakfast. His wife is feeling better and comes to visit at lunchtime. He eats a bit better and feels calmer. That evening, he falls asleep and sleeps heavily through the night.

On Tuesday, Charlie is better rested and appears calmer and more content through the day. Wednesday is also uneventful. On Thursday, however, Charlie becomes upset when the shower he is given is too cold. The water is eventually warmed, but he is combative for the rest of his bathing and dressing. He is out of sorts during the day. His wife's visit brings a temporary calming effect, but the commotion of staff leaving at the end of the day shift makes him upset because he feels he needs to go to work. The staff's attempts to convince him to stay are met with further agitation. He is again restless at night and has insufficient sleep.

On Friday, Charlie is reluctant to get out of bed when asked. He is tired and wants to sleep in. The staff get him up amid much resistance and finally get him washed and dressed. In the lounge, he falls asleep in the chair. His wife comes to visit and takes him around the grounds in a wheelchair. He is calmer after she leaves and again has a night of catching up on lost sleep. Saturday and Sunday pass without incident. His family sees him daily. The following Monday, he also appears calm as the day begins.

If we were to construct a graph of Charlie's behavior over the week, we would see that it does not follow a regular daily rhythm. However, a careful review of the week reveals that he is very sensitive to the social dynamic of the nursing home environment. By doing an observation log, many factors can be identified that have affected his demeanor—interactions with staff, unfamiliar care partners, excessive or inadequate stimulation, family absences, and attempts to force his pattern of sleeping and waking.

Creating an observation log can suggest many interventions to improve Charlie's care environment and his well-being. However, many people have less tolerance for simply observing such mood fluctuations and are quick to respond with medication. This is illustrated in

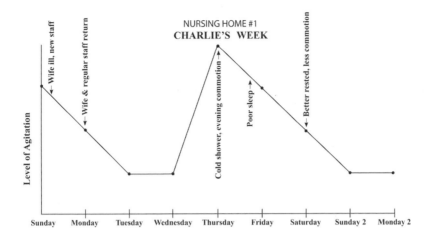

Level of Agitation

NURSING HOME #1
CHARLIE'S WEEK

Wife ill, new staff

Wife & regular staff return

Cold shower, evening commotion →

Poor sleep →

← Better rested, less commotion

Sunday   Monday   Tuesday   Wednesday   Thursday   Friday   Saturday   Sunday 2   Monday 2

how the staff responds in the following description of the same week in a different nursing home.

> In Nursing Home #2, the nursing staff does not see that the absence of Charlie's wife and the unfamiliar staff are contributing to his anxiety. They are quick to report Charlie's Sunday agitation to the medical doctor on call. An antipsychotic pill is started at a low dose. Charlie sleeps well on Monday night and has two more quiet days. In this home, however, the quiet and calm days are not noted to be related to the return of his wife and the regular staff members. Instead, because the staff views him as needing medication, the calm days are seen as a positive effect from the drug.
>
> On Thursday, the agitation returns, due to the environmental factors of the cold shower and commotion of the staff leaving in the afternoon. However, this home is not logging behavior patterns; it is simply reacting to what is observed. By Friday, staff members have reported to a doctor that "the medication worked for a couple of days, but now he's getting 'revved up' again." The doctor responds by doubling the dose of medication.
>
> The weekend progresses calmly, and the report on the following Monday is that Charlie is doing well on his medication.

We have seen a week in the life of Charlie as lived in two different nursing homes. His experience in both homes was exactly the same. But in Nursing Home #1, social and environmental patterns were observed that will impact future care planning, and in Nursing Home

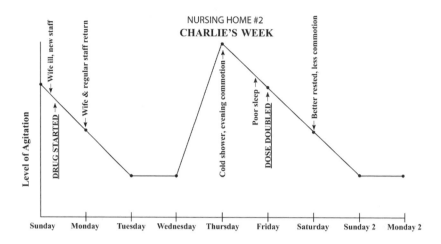

#2, he was put on psychotropic medication that was erroneously credited with producing his calm demeanor at the end of the week.

Other Medications

An examination of the other classes of drugs used for behavioral symptoms reveals the same constellation of weak results, significant risks, and lingering questions about exactly what the drug is doing. The Sink et al. review of 2005 did not find much evidence for *any* class of medication.

We have seen that the use of medication for behavioral expressions is far less effective and far more dangerous than most people realize. We have also seen that, in spite of this, their use has rapidly increased over the past several years. How can we explain such a seemingly contradictory trend?

As the number of people living with dementia continues to increase, our broken model of care becomes more apparent in the increasing levels of distress that these people experience. The biomedical view of dementia puts the focus on the disease, and, as such, the logical remedy is some sort of medical treatment. Because behavioral expressions are often viewed as pathology, the natural response is to medicate in an effort to do something.

Care professionals and family members want to see this approach work. All parties want to see dementia as something that can be treated and maybe someday cured. The development of the biomedical view of dementia, according to Cheston and Bender (1999), is part of an attempt to "remove aging from the realm of nature and place it within the realm of science" (p. 280). Everyone fears dementia, and treating the person with pills also treats everyone's fears that the disorder may not be within our control.

Cheston and Bender (1999) also assert that the biomedical view

> is antagonistic to models of social change that imply that there is a reality greater than the individual's brain. Moreover, in a culture that is always in a hurry, the much faster relief that drugs offer is of great importance. Medication can offer an apparently quick way to calm people down and lift their mood or to keep a ward seemingly calm and orderly. The fact that many of these drugs have side effects is often played down or ignored. (p. 276)

Practitioners prescribe these drugs because they do not have a more effective alternative. Most are quite aware of the pitfalls of these drugs but simply do not have a better pill to use. This is the essence of the problem: *we are only looking for a better pill*. But what if the best approach is not a pill?

Cautionary Tales

Further evidence that we need a new approach comes from the many "awakenings" we have seen in people who have been able to stop taking these medications. In fact, these awakenings can be so dramatic that we should be asking ourselves another important question: What other effects of these medications may go unrecognized and be potentially devastating?

To this end, I will share a few remarkable stories, which I will call (with apologies to Geoffrey Chaucer) *The Cautionary Tales*.

The Mason's Tale

Mason, as in Dr. Amy Mason, one of my practice partners, has always been very proactive in minimizing unnecessary medications. Her patient, Jean, arrived in late August after a long hospitalization. Jean was 77 and had had worsening memory over the past year, punctuated by intermittent episodes of increased confusion. She also had trouble walking and had fallen 2 months earlier, fracturing a lumbar vertebra. She was seen in the hospital emergency room and, after returning home with her usual prescriptions plus a pain pill, became more lethargic and could not eat.

Jean returned to the hospital and was found to have a

dangerously low sodium level in her blood. This was caused by a combination of medications that affected her ability to excrete water and also prevented her bladder from emptying. She was treated with a special IV solution and was given a catheter to empty the bladder until it regained function. However, due to reports of "suspiciousness," the hospital staff also started her on the antipsychotic pill risperidone.

Although her medical condition stabilized, Jean began to have worsening problems with her gait and balance in the hospital. She became more confused, her muscles became more rigid, and she fell. Jean's blood tests were now normal and a scan of the brain did not show any new problem. She was transferred to a rehabilitation unit but was unable to clear her confusion or walk independently. She was then moved to St. John's Home for long-term care. She was also scheduled to see a neurologist for "possible Parkinson's disease."

When Dr. Mason first met her, Jean had a great deal of word-finding difficulty and could not remember the details of her recent illness and hospitalization. She also had a fair amount of stiffness and a rigidity of the limbs similar to that seen in Parkinson's disease. However, similar symptoms can be seen as a side effect of risperidone. Dr. Mason did not see any evidence of delusional symptoms, and she rapidly reduced the risperidone dose over several days, and then stopped it completely.

A few days after she moved to St. John's Home, Jean went to see the neurologist, who recommended starting a new medication for her Parkinson-like symptoms. However, Dr. Mason elected to give her more time off the risperidone before adding any new medication. Jean was seen by our consulting psychiatrist $2\frac{1}{2}$ weeks after stopping the drug, and he noted her to be "stylish" in her appearance, with very good rapport and no word-finding difficulty. Her family found her level of interaction to be more like it had been 6 months earlier.

Four weeks after she arrived at St. John's, Jean had no further rigidity in her limbs. Another trial of physical therapy was ordered. This time, she improved nicely—in a matter of days she was able to walk 250 feet and got in and out of her bed and chair independently. On October 3, she was discharged to an assisted living apartment, 6 weeks after she had come to our nursing home for "long-term" care.

Little Emma's Tale

Little Emma was well under 5 feet tall. She was part of the growing population of people with Down syndrome who have lived into their 60s. Down syndrome produces a cognitive decline in middle age that is pathologically identical to Alzheimer's disease.

Emma's devoted siblings cared for her for many years after her parents passed away. Her nieces and nephews were very affectionate and used to "rough-house" with her from time to time. However, Emma did not always know when gentle hitting was an appropriate form of play or when it was overly rough. Her family reported that she also began to wander and "get into things" at home. She was placed on the antipsychotic drug haloperidol for her "aggression" and other behavioral symptoms.

Emma came to St. John's Home several months later after the family could no longer care for her. She had become unable to walk, and she barely spoke. She was incontinent and needed help with meals and all personal care. When I first saw her, she was lethargic, nonverbal, and stiff as a board.

Now that she was in an environment where we could investigate her symptoms carefully, I discontinued the haloperidol. She gradually became more alert, and her rigidity diminished. One day, when an aide was passing her door, she heard a bizarre noise and looked inside. There was Emma, laughing and jumping up and down on her bed like a kid at a pajama party!

Emma was with us for nearly 2 years before her dementia progressed to the point where she could no longer thrive. During that time, she roamed the floor independently, enjoyed her meals, and spoke and interacted with everyone she encountered. She also spent a few mornings each week at a day program in the community for adults with disabilities.

Emma could be rambunctious, and she occasionally strolled into rooms where she was not welcome. She would occasionally strike out at care partners, not realizing that it was inappropriate to do so. The staff developed a behavioral approach that gave Emma a "time out" in her room on such occasions; she would invariably emerge after a few minutes, say "sorry," and be on her way.

Whenever concerns were raised about her behavior, the staff repeatedly rallied to adjust the care plan to keep Emma from being moved to another location. No antipsychotics were used again.

The Dancer's Tale

Anitra had been living a marginal existence for some time. She shared an apartment in the city with a gentleman friend, but both were aging and losing their cognitive abilities. Her friend tried to support her but was increasingly inattentive to her forgetfulness. Late one night, she was found wandering the streets and was unable to tell the police where she lived.

Anitra was brought to the local hospital emergency room, and after it was determined that there were no acute medical problems, it was decided that her living situation was unsafe. She was moved to St. John's Home. Although her friend continued to make periodic visits, Anitra had difficulty adjusting to the home. She was usually very calm and conversant during the day, but it was very difficult to keep her in bed at night.

After being helped to bed, usually between 8 and 9 p.m., Anitra would often try to get up again. What followed was a cat-and-mouse game with the nurses, which lasted long into the night shift. She required almost constant attention due to her inability to settle down and stay in bed. Sleep medications either were ineffective or left her lethargic into the following day. She even fell and had a fracture not long after she came to St. John's, but this did not slow her attempts to get out of bed at night.

Eventually, some of Anitra's estranged relatives located her and came to visit her. In taking a more thorough history, her nighttime problems were mentioned to the family. They informed us that Anitra had been a Las Vegas showgirl for most of her adult life. Apparently, she had rarely gone to bed before 4 a.m. for decades.

With this knowledge, the staff stopped trying to put Anitra to bed in the early evening and let her stay up into the night shift. She was set up in the lounge with a television show or soft music, and she interacted with the staff when they passed. Her demeanor improved, and she resumed her lifelong habit of "late to bed and late to rise."

We were able to obtain a stunning portrait of the "dancer" Anitra, which she kept in her room. Her care partners would dance with her as long as she was able to maintain some degree of balance. Anitra's dementia progressed, and nearly 2 years after she came to live with us she passed away peacefully and medication-free.

Phair and Good (1998) remind us that "people with dementia should be empowered to find their own balance between activity and wakefulness, rest and sleep." They add that "care professionals should adapt the needs of the [environment] around them, ensuring that they do not inflict their own standards on the people in their care" (p. 94).

The foregoing stories are representative of the many awakenings that we have seen in people who have been taken off antipsychotic drugs and given a more individualized approach to care. Should behavioral symptoms reappear, we need to investigate them and determine the best response. On rare occasion, a drug may be restarted at an equal or lower dose, but the vast majority of people whom we take off these medications are able to stay off. Several studies have shown that with targeted psychosocial interventions, antipsychotic medication could be stopped in most people with a history of agitation without worsening their symptoms (Avorn et al., 1992; Ballard et al., 2008; Cohen-Mansfield et al., 1999; Van Reekum et al., 2002).

Beyond the realm of antipsychotic drugs, however, there are other medications used for behavioral symptoms. Antiseizure medications such as valproic acid are used as mood stabilizers. They have also been considered to be safer alternatives in older people with dementia and agitation. In fact, St. John's Home was a study site for these medications (Porsteinsson, Tariot, Erb, and Gaile, 1997). Of course, I have a pair of *Cautionary Tales* for this drug as well, and they are probably the most amazing stories I have to tell.

Joanie's and Julia's Tales

When Joanie came to St. John's Home in February 2003, she was relatively young at 69 but doing poorly in her own home. She had undergone surgery for spinal stenosis in the past, but she continued to have pain and limited mobility. She had become increasingly weak and had difficulty walking. She had also developed difficulty with her memory. Her only other medical history was a seizure disorder that had been inactive for many years, and for which she took the antiseizure medicine valproic acid. She was transferred to St. John's Home after being hospitalized for a bladder infection complicated by dehydration.

When I first met Joanie, I noticed that she had a very flat expression and an emotionless manner of speech. She seemed apathetic, and our attempts to help her stand and walk were unsuccessful. She was soon discontinued from physical therapy and remained unable to walk, transferring from bed to chair with a mechanical lift.

In spite of her obvious inability to get around and manage independently, Joanie repeatedly asked me why she couldn't go back home again. I would patiently explain to her that, because she couldn't stand and walk, she would require 24-hour assistance, which was not available to her at home.

Her Folstein Mini-Mental State Exam score was only 13/30, indicating a moderately severe level of dementia. I recall noting in the chart that I felt she conversed better than most people do with that score, and she looked "more like someone who would score an 18 or 19." There was no doubt in my mind that she had dementia, but I wondered if her flat expression indicated some underlying depression. However, a trial of an antidepressant drug didn't seem to make any difference.

Our consulting psychiatrist was contacted and he felt that her apathy was due to her dementia, possibly an uncommon type targeting the frontal lobe of her brain, which helps regulate emotions. Her care plan continued unchanged, another trial of physical therapy failed, and she spent the next year in a similar state of health and function. Her questions about going home continued, and I continued to respond as before. My responses were somewhat vague because I didn't want to erase all of her hope, but I knew that she was not likely to improve.

In March 2004, after more than a year at St. John's Home, I was seeing Joanie for a routine exam. Her daughter was visiting from Texas, and she mentioned to Linda Reid, the nurse manager, that Joanie had not had a seizure in many years. Linda asked me if Joanie really needed to keep taking the valproic acid. I consulted a neurologist, who felt that a trial off the medication would be reasonable; the risk of having another seizure was minimal, since she didn't drive or even walk. We carefully tapered her off the medication and she remained seizure-free. But that's only part of the story.

Something remarkable happened. Joanie asked to see me a couple of months after her medication had been stopped. She wanted to have another trial of physical therapy to try to stand because she hated using the lift to get out of bed. I didn't expect any improvement after 15 months without any walking, but I told her I would ask Marian, her therapist, to see her once again. I was surprised when Marian said that Joanie had shown some improved strength and that she wanted to work with her for a week or two.

Over the next several weeks, Joanie not only stood, she began to walk again—first a few steps, then around the floor, then even longer distances. Her demeanor didn't change greatly, but she seemed more alert and cognizant, so out of curiosity I repeated her Folstein test in the Fall of 2004. She scored a perfect 30/30!

Joanie gradually continued to improve, and on May 15, 2005, she was discharged from St. John's Home to an independent apartment in the community. She had been at our nursing home for over 2 years and had not stood or walked for well over half of that time.

As this miraculous recovery progressed, we pored over her records to try to find the event to which we could ascribe her transformation. We examined blood tests and medication changes, and we re-read all of the other entries in her chart during the weeks leading up to the therapy sessions. Only one possible cause was found: the discontinuation of her valproic acid medication. And yet, she had never appeared sedated or otherwise affected by the pill, and her blood tests were always in the normal range.

I was unable to find any verification of this theory, but the following year, at a Geriatric Fellows' luncheon conference, one of the doctors presented a remarkably similar case of what he called "a previously unreported side effect of valproic acid." Now there were two cases, and I knew that it was no coincidence.

Valproic acid is commonly used, not only for seizures and depressive illnesses, but also for behavioral symptoms of dementia. How many others might be affected by the drug? It is alarming to think that a medication caused a woman to spend over 2 years in a nursing home in a state of disability—one that probably never would have occurred if the pill had been stopped earlier.

Another elder at St. John's, Julia, lived with us for over 7 years. She had a history of dementia as well as bipolar disease. She had also been taking valproic acid for many years as a mood stabilizer. Her dementia was significant when she arrived, to the point where her responses to my questions were vague—rarely more than a word or two. She would occasionally offer a complaint of pain but otherwise said little. I attributed this to her advancing dementia accompanied by a language barrier (she was born in Ukraine). She spent almost all of her time in her room with the television on, rarely paying attention to it or interacting with others. She did this for years.

About 6 years into her stay with us, I decided that since Julia's dementia seemed quite advanced, and since she had shown no signs of any mood problems during those years, it would be reasonable to try her off the valproic acid. Though not as dramatic as Joanie's transformation, I was surprised at a visit 2 months later to see Julia alert, smiling, and answering my questions accurately in very fluent English. She still had features of moderate dementia but was much more interactive, and her memory was clearly improved.

One day, she stopped me to tell me that her right leg was hurting more due to her arthritis. I told her that I would increase her pain medicine and check with the nurses after the weekend to see if it was helping. In the past I had found her to be completely unaware of the day or date. But the following Monday, Julia said to her nurse, "Tell Doctor Power that my leg is feeling better now. He will be checking with you today."

Her nurse also told me that one day during a family visit, when a breathing treatment was being given to Julia for her asthma, her daughter asked the nurse when she would come back to take the mask off. Julia shook her head, pointed at the clock, and stated firmly: "No! Fifteen minutes! I will do it!"

One day, Julia presented to one of her nurses, Debbie Calhoun, a gift for Debbie's daughter, which she had instructed her family to buy. She had recalled Debbie saying that her daughter's birthday was approaching and had planned this surprise.

To hear these stories after nearly 6 years of minimally responsive interaction amazed me and reminded me of Joanie's story. Once again, the only connection we found was the discontinuation of the medication. And once again, there was no outward sign of sedation, and her drug levels and other blood tests had been normal throughout her stay.

Julia died peacefully in the Spring of 2009. We all tried to give her the best care possible. It is sobering to think, however, of how much ability she was deprived of to fully engage with life over those 6 years—because of a pill.

The use of medication assumes that changing the chemistry of the brain will affect complex behavioral expressions in a positive manner. But the studies do not bear this out, and these stories should give us pause. So what else can be done?

In order to understand the framework of an *experiential* approach, I will next examine the underlying system of care that leads to the use of these medications in the first place. This larger entity, *the institutional model of care*, must be fully understood and then dismantled in order to find a new path to growth and fulfillment for those who live with dementia.

CHAPTER 3

"I Have a Feeling We're Not in Kansas Anymore"

Experiencing the Institutional Model

A Brief History of the Modern Nursing Home

The model that characterizes most U.S. nursing homes today has its roots in the Medicare and Medicaid Act of 1965. Faced with a growing population of aging Americans, Congress enacted legislation to help pay for their health care needs. In addition to providing medical coverage for people who are elderly, poor, and chronically disabled, they recognized the need to help more Americans finance long-term care. Because a large social program for elder care was likely to meet with public resistance, long-term care was tied into this medical reimbursement program.

The good news is that many people who once would have been relegated to the nation's poorhouses can now receive nursing home care. But this benefit comes at a steep price, for the model created by this system has turned nursing homes into medical institutions.

If reimbursement of long-term care is tied into a medical insurance program, then it becomes dependent upon medical diagnoses and treatments. Thus the lives of people in nursing homes have become medicalized, and the amount of reimbursement for their care depends on the diagnoses that they carry and the medical procedures that are carried out on their behalf. This system produces several results that are counterproductive to good care for our elders.

The first and most basic result is that *aging is viewed as pathology*, and the care of our frail elders revolves around their illnesses and functional limitations, rather than their individual identities and strengths. The result is a paternalistic, protective environment, where most of our efforts are directed toward what Dr. William Thomas refers to as "mitigated aging" (2004, p. 84).

Another result of this system is that interventions that provide reimbursement dollars are favored over those that do not. This puts the *emphasis on medical treatment* as the dominant feature of the nursing home. The tasks of the various staff members are prioritized around the need to perform these treatments, and interactions that are more holistic and that tend to the human spirit are frowned upon as a poor use of time and resources. This system also has a counterpart in community-based care and in the types of resources that are available to people living at home.

The emphasis on medical treatment also leads to a *backward system of financial incentives for care*. Consider, for example, the problem of pressure sores. Everyone agrees that these are not a good outcome. However, the reimbursement paid for daily treatment of a pressure sore is relatively high. If the home is successful in healing the pressure sore, subsequent reimbursement drops because the daily treatments are no longer being administered.

Imagine for a moment how nursing home care might change if a system were created that rewarded *wellness instead of illness*. Imagine how it would be if the financial payout were the same for medical procedures as for the interactions that build nurturing relationships, validate elders for who they are, and help them to engage with life. If a home were paid for the number of high-risk people who were successfully cared for *without* developing pressure sores, how differently would resources be allocated?

Moving In

Now that we have reviewed the history of the institutional model, let's experience it through the eyes of the elder who arrives there to live. A move to a traditional nursing home is accompanied by a multitude of losses. Some of these are material losses, but many are not.

First among the material losses is the loss of one's personal living space and the many possessions that must be left behind. These possessions may have provided comfort (a favorite chair), validation (mementos of lifetime accomplishments), identity and connectedness (photos and other keepsakes), or relaxation and enjoyment (a garden, a piano, or a favorite hobby). A beloved pet may be left behind. There is also the loss of daily communion with a spouse or other close family members. Many such moves include the loss of a car and with it the feeling of independence it symbolizes in our society.

Nonmaterial losses can be even more devastating to the individual faced with such a move. There is loss of privacy in a new world of double rooms, shared bathrooms, and communal lounging and eating areas. Dignity can be lost through infantilizing treatment by caregivers, transporting semiclad people to shower rooms, and making inappropriate comments in public areas. Worse still is the loss of control over almost every aspect of daily life, from deciding when to get up in the morning and when to eat, to having meaningful input into one's daily schedule, activity choices, or any other expression of individuality.

Finally, the institution often strips life of meaning for our elders. This meaning resides not only in our possessions and treasured objects, but also in the way each of us engages with the world around us. Traditional nursing homes erode meaning by standardizing daily routines; using generic approaches to meals, activities, and therapies; and creating a world in which the elders are dependent upon their caregivers and can no longer give care to others.

In a study of homeless individuals, Carboni (1990) identified several losses that characterized this group of people, including loss of identity, meaningful activity, connectedness, personal space, privacy, and security. She then studied residents of traditional nursing homes and found the same characteristic losses as were seen in the homeless. It is as if we have created an additional 1.8 million homeless people nationwide by placing them in traditional nursing homes!

The result of all these losses can be nothing less than a grief reaction, and this grief can be profound. It can even be fatal. Haven't we all seen elders who seem to "give up" after moving into a nursing home? Haven't we all heard people say, "I don't know why God doesn't just take me!"? What they are saying is, "Life no longer holds any meaning for me."

In his book *Man's Search for Meaning* (1959), psychiatrist Viktor Frankl wrote of his imprisonment in two Nazi concentration camps. He found that the prisoners who could not find meaning in their daily tasks became most despondent and most likely to provoke the guards to kill them.

Unfortunately, the institutional model does not recognize this grief for what it encompasses. Often, it is diagnosed as a "behavior problem." At best, the individual is identified as having an "adjustment disorder." But this is no disorder. Who among us would not find such a transition difficult? (In his book, Frankl also famously stated that "an abnormal reaction to an abnormal situation is normal behavior" [p. 38].)

This grief is compounded when a person's coping and adaptive skills are further compromised by dementia. Society allows us a year to grieve the loss of a loved one, yet how often do we rush to medicate the grief that accompanies institutionalization?

Keep in mind that most people admitted to nursing homes did not plan their move ahead of time. Rather, they were sent to the hospital for an acute illness or injury and then told they could not return home. Few people have time to plan for this major life transition that lies in their immediate future. A recent audit of 190 people admitted to St. John's Home in Rochester, New York, for long-term care over a year showed that 67.4% came here directly after a hospital stay. Another 22.2% came from another nursing home or assistive living community. Only 10.5% came directly from their homes.

A Parable

The story I am about to relate was written by Dr. William Thomas for his allegorical tale, *In the Arms of Elders* (2006). With his permission, I have altered the wording slightly in this parable of elder care to enhance its applicability to dementia.

The Story of Khalid the Kind

Long ago, when the people were still new to this world, a man lived with his family at the southern edge of the Great Desert in the village of Tum-Bak-Tee. Like his father and his father before him, he was a desert trader. Twice each year, once in the Spring and once in the Autumn, the trader would pack up his wares and harness his camel for the trek north to Mar-Kasha. Because he was a man of modest means and could not afford a caravan, he traveled alone.

Journey after journey, year after year, all was well. Then, one year, things went terribly wrong. As was his custom, the trader ventured north in the Spring and, for the first 8 days, made steady progress on the road to Mar-Kasha. On the morning of the 9th day, however, a wind began to dance across the desert. At first it was little more than a breeze, but it came from the west. The trader knew well that many deadly storms had grown from just such a wind as this.

The wind gained strength, lifting the scalding sand into the air. The trader's fear grew. Then the wind became an enormous black cloud of angry sand. It bore down on the trader and tore at his flesh. It lashed his faithful camel like a thousand braided whips. The beast stopped and refused to advance. The trader tumbled from his wailing beast and crawled to a nearby dune. There, he dug a pit and crawled into its depth. Above him, the wind howled its unending song of fury and pain.

By the time the morning light came, the storm was spent, and the trader unearthed himself from his hiding place. He searched frantically for his supplies and his camel. They were lost. He looked for the road to Mar-Kasha. It, too, was lost, erased by the power of the storm. He scrambled up the nearest dune and surveyed his surroundings, but all he saw was a boundless ocean of sand. Thinking a different view might give him some hope, he descended from that dune and climbed another. The scene was the same. All the while, the sun rose higher in the sky. Soon, the trader's tongue cried for water, but he had none. His stomach pinched with hunger, but there was no food. That night, he shivered under the desert's cold canopy of stars.

When morning came again, his lips were cracked and his tongue was swollen. He thought of his family and how much they needed him. He forced himself to climb one more dune. When his eyes found only sand, he knew that his life was nearly over.

What the unfortunate trader did not know—in fact, what he could not know—was that the oasis of Khalid the Kind lay just 1 hour's walk to the east. Khalid's Oasis was blessed with the finest, purest water in the desert, and Khalid was famous for possessing the most generous heart the desert had ever known. Khalid regularly rode the dunes in search of the lost and the forsaken.

Just as the trader prepared to close his eyes for the last time, Khalid discovered him. Khalid climbed down from his mount. He picked the trader up in his powerful arms, laid him across his camel's back, and rode swiftly home.

Back at the Oasis, Khalid offered the trader water. The man drank deeply. Again and again he drank. At last, the water had answered his thirst, and the trader was able to speak. "You must be Khalid the Kind," he croaked. "You have saved me when Death held his hand upon my throat."

Khalid answered, "It was the will of God that you should live. Now drink; drink more, for surely you've not taken enough."

"I am grateful to you, but I have taken my fill of water. Now I feel a great hunger, and I'm tired. Might I have something to eat and a place to lie down?"

"Food? How can you think of food?" Khalid thundered. "Not so long ago, you were nearly dead of thirst. Drink!" With that, Khalid held up the skin of water. The trader turned his head away, and the water spilled to the ground. This action convinced Khalid that the desert sun had addled the trader's mind. Wasting no time, Khalid again picked up the trader. With the trader firmly in his grip, he waded into the cool, fresh water of the spring.

Once he reached its deepest spot, Khalid began to dunk the trader's head into the water. The man thrashed and struggled, choking and gasping. He swallowed great gulps of fresh water. Over and over, Khalid plunged the trader's head into the water. The man began to struggle less. Khalid was pleased with this.

But soon the man's strength began to wane drastically. This alarmed Khalid greatly, so he held him under for longer and longer periods to ensure the man would drink.

In the end, the trader's strength dwindled to nothing. Death took him. Tears streaked the face of Khalid the Kind as he carried the trader's still warm body from the spring to a place just outside of the Oasis. There Khalid dug a shallow grave and laid the man to rest. He said the necessary prayers and covered him with sand and stones. This was not the first body laid to rest by Khalid the Kind.

When he was finished, Khalid returned to the Oasis. There, he harnessed his camel and rode out into the desert heat again, muttering as he went, "Water, they must have water" (pp. 118–121).

Like all of the parables in Thomas's book, the story of Khalid the Kind holds many lessons. First and foremost is that Khalid represents the medical model of elder care. Our treatments are the water that Khalid continued to force on the unlucky traveler, which ultimately caused his demise.

However, let's not rush to condemn the doctors alone for overmedicating our elders. After all, who is it that calls them on the phone to say, "Mr. Smith is out of control—we need something!"? Doctors, nurses, aides, social workers, even family members have bought into the ill-conceived notion that better care simply means more medical treatment. As we have seen, even our reimbursement system perpetuates this medicalization of care.

Was Khalid a bad man? Not at all—he was Khalid the Kind, with the most generous heart in the desert! Nor was he stupid. He was simply stuck in an old paradigm that kept him from seeing the danger of his well-intended efforts to save the trader.

A second lesson from the story is that it reminds us of the way most people come to nursing homes. Most people are traveling along as they always have, perhaps hanging on to independence by a tenuous thread, but hanging on nonetheless. Then the unexpected "storm" arrives—a broken hip, a stroke, a severe infection. They emerge into an unfamiliar landscape: the nursing home. The road back home is lost and they are weak and often near death.

For people with dementia, this landscape is even more confusing. Like the trader roaming the desert, they begin to wander the halls, looking for something familiar. In the medical model, this is often seen as a sign of pathology, rather than an attempt to find meaning and familiarity in new surroundings. For those who cannot walk, panic sets in; alternatively, people may withdraw and, like the trader, they may lose the strength to go on.

The needs of frail elders are many, as are those of people with dementia. But all too often, these needs are seen as a lack of "water"—medication, that is. One of the greatest failures of the biomedical model is our tendency to treat the body when people suffer from diseases of the spirit. Instead of adopting a more holistic approach that looks at emotional and spiritual needs, we pile on the medications, often with disastrous results.

A third lesson is highlighted by the sentences I have added to the original tale. Initially, as Khalid holds the man's head under water, his struggles lessen and Khalid is pleased. How often do we interpret the sedating effects of medication as a sign of a positive response? Have we brought our elders more happiness and well-being or have we simply made them quieter? And is that "quietude" a prelude to a more serious drug complication?

Inside the Institution

The legendary actress Mae West once said, "Marriage is a great institution, but I'm not ready for an institution yet." On the subject of institutional living, most of us would agree as well. The traditional nursing home of the past half century is very much an institution in many ways. However, an institution is more than a structure—it is a living, breathing entity. Thomas (2008) refers to it as "the dragon sleeping in the corner," always ready to be awakened whenever care decisions are being made.

To understand all that comprises this creature and its effect on elder care, we must examine three characteristics of the institutional nursing home—*physical, operational,* and *interpersonal.*

If we think of an institution as a living entity, then the differences between a home and an institution revolve around whether each component serves the individuals who live there or the larger creature. Our *physical* images of institutions usually revolve around dark, cheerless buildings with tile floors and walls painted some unpleasant shade of green. But, as we will see, a bright cheery-looking facility can also be very institutional.

In order to serve the dragon, the facility is constructed with efficiency and cost savings in mind. Thus a centrally located nurses' station is a hallmark of most nursing homes. Metal carts are wheeled down the long corridors, bringing medications to each room in an efficient manner. Many people live in double rooms, sometimes even triples or quads, built to maximize use of square footage. Bathrooms are shared, and narrow hospital-style beds are separated only by a thin "privacy curtain." Large fluorescent lights give maximum illumination to the beds, often glaring into the eyes of the occupants in the process.

There is little space for personal belongings in each room and the use of one's personal furniture is often discouraged, as it is more efficient to keep standardized furnishings in the room through a succession of occupants. Gathering areas tend to be places where people can be herded together in front of a television set, which is often tuned to a station few care to watch. Multistory buildings make efficient use of land but require elders to use elevators, denying most of them direct or easy access to the outside world.

It is not unusual to see 40 or more people living in one area, which can create a chaotic social environment, particularly for those with dementia. Hallways are long and may require a walk of 100 feet or more to get to the dining room. Many elders become *functionally disabled* because their environment requires more effort to navigate than their home did.

Staff time is made efficient by the use of call bells and intercoms, which can sound frighteningly loud in the speakers over one's bed. These, and the use of bed and chair alarms, create a level of background noise that can heighten feelings of anxiety even in people without cognitive impairment.

I am sure that the reader can think of many other physical features of the institutional nursing home. It is essential to realize that *none of the features just described can be found in anyone's home.* Keep in mind that many nursing homes undergo extensive remodeling, but they keep most or all of these features. The carpets may be new and bright, the furniture may sparkle, but the nurses' stations, call bells, double rooms, and med carts all remain because the remodeling is done according to the institutional dragon's needs, not those of the individuals who live there. As will be discussed in detail later, this is important because much of the free-floating anxiety that accompanies dementia in the nursing home is related to these physical and environmental characteristics.

Some nursing homes have succeeded in creating a physical structure that does away with many of these features. Unfortunately, many of them may remain very institutional because the other two dimensions of the institution are ignored.

From an *operational* standpoint, institutional nursing homes are organized on a hospital model. Many of the physical features I have described relate to the traditional hospital layout, and the organizational structure follows a similar path. The hallmarks are a top-down decision-making hierarchy and the creation of separate departments to handle the various operational needs of the facility.

The decision-making structure looks like a corporate "family tree," with the board of directors and/or CEO at the top of the chart. Descending levels of authority occupy each successive row beneath. The visual impression of the organizational chart reflects the reality that the power increases the higher you go, and trouble generally flows downhill. At the bottom rung, if they are included at all, are the direct care staff. The elders living in the home and their families rarely make the chart.

This structure is rigid in both vertical and horizontal directions. Vertically, many decisions are made by directors and managers, even though the elders and hands-on staff may be primarily affected and have more intimate knowledge of their needs. Horizontally, there is often little interdepartmental communication and cooperation. Two rank-and-file workers from different departments may figure out a better way to accomplish a task, but they must each send the idea up their respective departmental ladders until their superiors can confer and decide if the idea has merit.

The segregation of tasks can actually create barriers to both efficiency and good care. St. John's CEO, Charlie Runyon, once described it to me succinctly: "In the institution, the tops of the dining room tables are cleaned by food service and the legs are cleaned by housekeeping."

As with the physical structure, the operational structure feeds the institutional dragon rather than the elders and those who care for them. Centralized services are felt to be more efficient; food is prepared in a central kitchen and distributed on trays at fixed mealtimes, people are wakened and bathed at times that reflect the needs of the staff instead of the elders, and a staff member may sidestep a problem that doesn't fit her compartmentalized job description.

This last aspect is particularly counterproductive to humanistic care because employees are taught to place tasks before people, and these tasks become the central focus of the job. The true customer has been lost in the pile of daily duties to be performed. Thus any attempt to transform the care environment is difficult because the employees see it as another task to add to the list they already have, and they feel there is not enough time to "do culture change."

Unfortunately, this resistance can be fostered by a hierarchical structure that often does not value the wisdom of its hands-on staff. This corps of people who do some of the most caring and compassionate work in elder care is underappreciated, even vilified in both nursing home and community-based care. The *2006–2007 Occupational Outlook Handbook* from the U.S. Department of Labor describes the job of the nursing assistant as follows: "Modest entry requirements, low pay, high physical and emotional demands, and lack of advancement opportunities characterize this occupation." Is it any wonder we have staff shortages in this critical area of need?

The Eden Alternative has a Golden Rule that states, "As management does unto staff, so shall staff do unto the elders." Unfortunately, in institutions, management creates a task-driven mindset that drives the behavior of the hands-on staff, and this mindset carries over to the bedside as well.

In writing about transformative nursing homes, Beth Baker

(2007) reflected on this attitude in her earlier career as a dialysis technician:

> A supervisor once chastised me for spending a few minutes talking with patients as I put them on the dialysis machine, a painful, stressful experience that involved having large needles stuck into their arms. "You're holding up production," he told me, without irony. (p. 66)

Social worker and consultant Cathy Unsino told me the story of a certified nursing assistant (CNA) who was reprimanded by her manager for taking time to escort a person outside after dinner to watch the sunset. To her credit, the CNA responded, "Well, *somebody* has to do it!"

Even though direct care workers spend the most time with the people who live in nursing homes, they are rarely consulted to share their thoughts and opinions. Formal care conferences and family meetings often occur without their valuable input.

At St. John's Home several years ago, we held focus group meetings with all staff to find out what they wanted to make their jobs better. There were certainly requests for higher pay; low pay is characteristic across all disciplines in long-term care. But the two top areas that were identified in our survey were *increased respect* and *better communication*, neither of which costs a penny.

In a culture in which the direct care workers are not valued, the greatest harm falls on the people they care for. It is impossible to have needs of the moment addressed when everyone is busy focusing on tasks and deferring to other departments or higher-ups. Furthermore, any attempt to express a need or to assert any individuality disrupts the well-oiled machinery of the institution and is viewed as a "problem." This concept is central in reframing our view of expressions of need in people with dementia.

Baker (2007) related a visit to a home in the Midwest, where a woman grabbed her hand and began shouting that the staff had tied her up and kidnapped her granddaughter. The experience left her shaken, but she later reflected on what she had seen:

> It was a brief window for me into how scary it would be to either live in this woman's world, or to be responsible for her care.
>
> I wondered, though, how much of her anger could be traced to her environment . . . [E]ven before I met the woman, I wanted to flee. Everything about the place felt wrong. You exited the elevator to face an imposing nurses' station. In the hallways, people sat in wheelchairs

with nothing going on to engage them. The atmosphere was stifling, and particularly distressing, as I knew this was a place with a good reputation. I felt I would go mad if I had to live there. Why should we expect anything different from residents, whatever their cognitive state? (p. 163)

The third facet of the institutional dragon is the *interpersonal* dimension. This is the least obvious, but potentially the most harmful. This is the *mindset* about aging and elder care that characterizes employees of any institution, and it affects their day-to-day interactions with each other and with the elders and their families. There are several components of this mindset.

First is the attitude perpetuated by the biomedical model that views elders as broken individuals and sees them primarily for their diseases and functional limitations, rather than as whole people. As a physician, I am aware that the typical "admission history and physical exam" is little more than finding out "What is wrong with you?" rather than "Who are you and what makes you a unique individual?" We will later explore how this view causes us to misinterpret behavioral clues and even provoke the behavioral symptoms we are trying to address.

Second, we view our roles from a paternalistic perspective. We have an operational structure that tells us that we know what is best—for those who report to us and, ultimately, for the elders in our care. This further disempowers individuals throughout the home.

A series of studies demonstrated very clearly that there is a tendency in nursing homes for staff members to ignore any attempts by the elders to participate more actively in their personal care (Baltes, 1988). This push for expedience actually perpetuates dependence among those same elders.

Therapeutic recreation specialist Mimi Bommelje told me a story about one of her favorite elders, Helen:

One day we were at the breakfast table. Helen reached for her glass of milk and someone swooped in, picked it up, and brought it to her lips. She promptly refused it. The staff member put it down and walked away.

She looked at me and said, "No one even gives you a chance around here!" I handed her the glass. She drank the milk.

A third attitude is the notion that aging is decline and that the function of a nursing home is protection and mitigation of that decline, rather than nurturing growth at all stages of life. With this comes a preference for risk avoidance and a one-dimensional view of elderhood and its potential.

Every time there is a problem to solve or a decision to make, the institutional dragon awakens and says, "Feed me!" More often than not, we obey. Why? Because dragons can scorch us. Those who don't follow the dictates of the institution could land in all kinds of trouble, from being "written up" to being "dressed down." Institutions thrive on efficiency and cost-effectiveness and do so by stifling diversity and individuality. Boring is good. If you make waves, you will be the one to suffer the consequences.

The mindset of the institutional nursing home is even more complicated because the dragon has friends whose influence is also felt throughout the organization. One of these is the "regulatory dragon," representing the federal and state oversight of long-term care. In many areas, the regulatory process places its focus on finding fault and punishing nursing homes, rather than acknowledging good work and educating homes that need help to improve. There is often an adversarial relationship between the home and the regulators; threats of financial penalties perpetuate the institutional mindset and discourage innovative approaches.

Regulators in turn can be ill served by their own superiors. One of the most irritating dictates is that regulators are not allowed to counsel nursing homes—only to tell them if what they are doing is out of compliance. The notion that regulators cannot mentor homes to become better without losing their objectivity as surveyors is an insult to their capabilities.

There is also the "liability dragon," which feeds on the fear of lawsuits, causing individual choice to be trampled in an environment that sometimes seems too risk averse even to breathe. Policies are drafted around the exception rather than the rule, and the freedoms of many are sacrificed to protect against the remote possibility that one person may suffer from an unwise decision.

A third member of the institutional dragon's circle is the "reimbursement dragon." This is the dragon that feeds our coffers, but only if our elders fulfill criteria that reinforce the medical model. There are many different reimbursement tools, but each assigns an acuity level to a nursing home resident that determines the person's daily rate of reimbursement. On the surface, this makes sense—the more complex someone's care is, the more it costs to provide that care—but there are several problems with this system.

One problem is the inequity within the system itself. Is a person who needs physical therapy or a daily dressing change harder to care for than a person who can walk independently but who is frequently agitated and distressed? Often not, but the system will pay far more to care for the first person than the second. Treatments are always valued more highly than time and caring.

Another problem with the current reimbursement system is that people whose conditions improve are moved to a lower reimbursement category, so that a nursing home is "rewarded" for its excellent care with a pay cut. This is how the reimbursement dragon helps his friends—by keeping us in a mindset that favors medical interventions for illness over promotion of wellness.

An example of this faulty system is that of a person recently transferred from the hospital. If this person's acute illness and hospitalization have left him weak and delirious, malnourished, incontinent, and dependent in his activities of daily living, he receives a high reimbursement score. If the nursing home gives him excellent care by restoring his nutritional balance, clearing his delirium, and providing therapy to improve his functional ability and continence, his score will drop and the home is "rewarded" with a drop in reimbursement.

In other words, we reward illness, frailty, and functional dependence while punishing the homes that improve the lots of their elders through good care. Imagine a school system in which teachers are paid more for the students who fail their classes, or a community whose police are given a pay cut when the crime rate falls. Welcome to long-term care.

———————

One of the people at our home, Marty, has severe Lewy body dementia. Many vexing behavioral expressions can accompany this atypical form of dementia. In Marty's case, he is given to tirades laced with profanity whenever he becomes uncomfortable or frustrated. The staff has worked to use a behavioral approach to address these outbursts with varying degrees of success, depending on the day and the situation.

One day, Marty's nurse, Theresa, was attending to him and he launched into one of his colorful litanies about the difficulties he had getting his needs met. Theresa said, "Why are you swearing at me, Marty? I thought we were friends!"

Marty shouted back, "I'm not swearing at you! I'm swearing at the institution!"

CHAPTER 4

"Abandon Hope"
A Deeper Look at Institutionalization

I HAVE EXAMINED THE PITFALLS of medication use for behavioral symptoms of dementia. I have also described the physical, operational, and interpersonal components that make up the institution, and the descriptions have shown that it is not a warm, welcoming place to live. It is clear that we need an alternative.

But before we can build this new model of care, it is important to look further into the infrastructure of the institutional model; there are some deeper flaws to be rooted out if a new approach is expected to truly transform the care of people who live with dementia.

Aging and Society

Our society has a rather dysfunctional view of aging that reaches far beyond our long-term care system. Nursing homes are not some aberration that suddenly appeared; nor were they simply created in their present form by nursing home operators. Rather, it is our *society's view of aging* that created the institutional model of nursing homes. In other words, if we don't like the way nursing homes operate, we all need to start by looking in the mirror.

To put this societal view simply, aging is decline. It is a slide from something good to something bad. The best we can do is to try to manage this decline to whatever degree we can.

When introducing in lectures his concept of *mitigated aging*— trying to make a bad thing less bad—Dr. William Thomas often likens the idea to "putting a scented air freshener on the back of the toilet." This is a far cry from viewing elders as leaders, historians, and wisdom keepers, as they were seen in most traditional societies. The source of this shift, according to Thomas, is the development of the "cult of adulthood."

In *What Are Old People For?*, Thomas (2004) takes a new look at the stages of human development, one that views growth as an interplay between two states: *doing* and *being*. Doing involves interacting with the world around you in a way that is visible or measurable. You can do a job, do your homework, or do a hobby. You can even "do lunch." Being, on the other hand, involves relating to the world in ways that are not necessarily visible or measurable. You can be in love, be reflective, be spiritual, or be imaginative.

As an infant, being is about all there is, beyond one's basic bodily functions. Small children gradually learn to do things, but every activity is still rich with being, and their imaginations can blossom during even the most mundane activities.

Children gradually acquire new doing skills through their schooling and then enter the turbulent transitional period of adolescence. The adolescent vacillates between states of doing and being "like a shutter that flaps back and forth in the wind" (Thomas, 2004, p. 122). Eventually, however, the adolescent moves into the stage of adulthood.

Adulthood is all about doing. It wasn't always that extreme, but it seems that our modern society values doing more than anything else. How long can you stand around at a social event before someone asks, "So, what do you do?" It's never, "Who are you? Tell me about yourself." We measure our worth by what we can visibly accomplish or produce. This is reflected in our increasingly long hours of work, filling our children's days with structured activities, avoiding activities that aren't goal directed, and devaluing anybody (including elders) who cannot do as much as we can.

Who are the elders that impress us in our modern society? The ones who still *do* a lot. Thus we are enthralled by the 90-year-old parachute jumper, the 88-year-old marathoner, the 85-year-old CEO. Once, in 2007, Thomas commented to me that "in our society the only good old person is an old person who looks and acts like a young person." If this is true, then frail elders in nursing homes must seem to have little value, and those with dementia least of all. Is it any wonder that we haven't built a better model of care for them?

Indeed, both the media and the government are frequently sounding alarms about the aging of the baby boomers and the "burden" it will place on our society. There is never a discussion of the gifts that such accumulated wisdom might bestow on a society that increasingly needs some "elder supervision."

In the nursing home, this cult of adulthood has many side effects. The overriding effect, as mentioned earlier, is the view of elders as primarily broken individuals. The diseases are real enough, but the institutional system uses those diseases to disempower and disconnect elders from autonomy and active engagement with life. In the care plan or the medical record, elders are reduced to a problem list of diseases and disabilities. They are described in a litany of what they can and cannot do: "Mr. Jones transfers with one assist. He ambulates with one assist and a gait belt. He is continent of bowel, incontinent of bladder. He eats independently after setup. He is dependent in other activities." But *who is he?*

Time and energy are devoted to coping with people's weaknesses, rather than cultivating their strengths. The resultant "care plan" often reduces the person's life to what Uman (1997) calls "a series of interventions" (p. 1026). This view also causes the institution to err on the side of "safety" in any decision, which often stifles growth and fulfillment. And, of course, the adults who work in the home always know best; they are the "whole, unbroken people."

The other effect of this attitude on nursing home relationships is that no interaction is considered legitimate or valuable unless it becomes a "therapy." Elders' days are filled with physical therapy, occupational therapy, speech therapy, recreation therapy, music therapy, pet therapy, plant therapy. Only doing, not being, counts in our society, so all of the being activities must be sanitized into preplanned, measurable, and billable therapies. It may look like a full day, but it is often devoid of spontaneity, variety, meaning, and joy.

If adulthood were the last stage of life, then this approach might make sense. And if adulthood is the pinnacle of life, then aging is a sad process indeed—a long, slow slide toward death. This explains the wealth of antiaging books and remedies that fill the shelves of shops, libraries, and bookstores.

But unlike most psychologists and philosophers, Thomas's stages of development do not end here. Instead, he proposes another transitional stage that mirrors the stage of adolescence. This he terms *senescence*, which is not senility, but rather a ripening. This is a stage in which adults reevaluate all that they are doing and begin to change their priorities. This is also a time when adults begin to synthesize years of life experience into wisdom.

This transition leads to the final stage, which Thomas calls *elderhood*. Elderhood is the most "being-rich" stage of life. Indeed, a study by Carstensen, Pasupathi, Mayr, and Nesselroade (2000) showed that older adults are happy more often than young adults, and they are unhappy for shorter periods of time. They place less value on material possessions and doing activities, and more value on relationships and spirituality. They also tend to view the world around them with a richer tapestry of thoughts and feelings, and they have a better understanding of complex emotional states such as poignancy.

Classical gerontology sees older adults as following one of two paths: continued activity or disengagement. This reflects a narrow adult view that values those who continue to do, to produce. More recently, the concept of gero-transcendence has been introduced. Carr (2005) describes this as "redefining the self in very old age with a new understanding of fundamental existential questions" (p. 82). This reflects the synthesis of wisdom and reminds us that not doing is not the same as disengaging.

The presence of a strong state of being is mirrored in elderhood and early childhood. This makes for good partnerships when day care centers can connect with elders in nursing homes.

> Lenny had severe dementia caused by repeated strokes, and he was unable to speak more than a few words. He was unable to walk or even propel his own wheelchair. But when the 2-year-olds from our child care center came to visit, the staff brought Lenny to the rec room, and a bond was formed with a boy named Andre.
>
> While the other children played or ran around, Andre sat quietly on Lenny's lap, watching the action. Neither of them was able to speak a great deal, but they seemed to gain comfort from this silent companionship. Occasionally, one of the staff members would push the wheelchair around the halls to give them a ride. I guess this was our way of interjecting a bit of doing into their being.

> I saw them together on several occasions—different ages, different races, but somehow very close, perhaps bound by their common need for being and their common inability to fully join the world of adults. Andre preferred sitting on Lenny's lap to joining in with the other children's games, and it was always hard to get him to leave.
>
> One day, I took a photo of the two of them together and gave it to Lenny. It stayed on his bedside shelf, a reminder of a source of companionship and contentment in his last days.

Imagine what would happen to the nursing home care plan if elders were viewed as complete adults who no longer have to be measured on the basis of what they can or cannot do, and who are fully valued simply for who they are. What would the care plan document look like then? What would their day be like? (We'll talk more about this later on.)

Well-Being and Personhood

Chapter 2 discussed the fact that drug intervention trials measure only negative symptoms rather than indices of well-being. So what exactly *is* well-being?

Many people have devised definitions or yardsticks for quality of life. Ready and Ott (2003) reviewed nine quality-of-life scales specifically applied to people with dementia. They concluded that the importance of considering quality of life (QOL) in dementia

> cannot be overstated . . . [H]ealthcare professionals might have a better ability to intervene to improve quality of life than to change other aspects of the disease. Assessment of QOL also has the important effect of calling attention to positive states and "personhood" in dementia, in contrast to most other measures of dementia that focus on deficits and pathology. (p. 7)

Most of these quality-of-life scales go beyond measures of negative behavioral symptoms to include positive attributes, such as social interaction, awareness of self, enjoyment of activities, self-esteem, and response to surroundings. Each scale is slightly different, but most are incomplete.

It is important to move beyond the concept of quality of life, which largely involves measurements still steeped in the biomedical model of wellness, and talk instead about well-being, which is a state that is not necessarily dependent on the presence or absence of disease or a person's activity level.

The Navajo Nation has a word, *hozho*, which means a state of being in harmony with nature. It is possible to be old, frail, or living with a chronic disease and yet still be in a state of harmony with the world. This is a concept of well-being that resonates with me. Can we break it down any further?

Fox et al. (2005) identified seven central domains of well-being: identity, growth, autonomy, security, connectedness, meaning, and joy. (Do these look familiar? They are nearly the same domains that Carboni found absent in homeless people and people in traditional nursing homes.) The authors admit, however, that well-being is elusive and highly subjective.

Kitwood and Bredin (1992) suggested 12 "indicators of well-being." However, it can be argued that some of them (such as initiation of social contact) may be impaired or absent in people with severe dementia. I believe that well-being should not be tied to what one can or cannot do; it should be possible to experience well-being regardless of one's cognitive or functional abilities.

Sabat (2001) refers to the more basic concept of a "glimmer of light still shining" (p. 109), reflecting the Spark of Life that Dementia Care Australia's program of the same name strives to rekindle in the eyes of people with dementia (see Resources). While this may sound unscientific, it is nevertheless a compelling and reliable sign that can be readily observed in those who are positively engaged with the world around them.

One of the most enduring statements on well-being is the hierarchy of needs described by Abraham Maslow in 1943. The pyramid describes Maslow's hierarchy, from the most basic needs at the bottom to more complex and integrative needs at the upper levels. At the bottom are the biological needs and the need for shelter and security. Above those is the need for love and connectedness, followed by achievement and self-esteem. Higher yet are the aesthetic needs for increased knowledge and exploration, and finally the need for self-actualization. Maslow considered self-actualization the key to a meaningful life. He cautioned that the higher levels of need cannot be satisfied if the lower needs remain unmet.

Is it necessary for everyone to strive to reach the top of the pyramid? Viktor Frankl would say so. As he described in *Man's Search for Meaning*, the ability to find meaning in life is a key to survival. We have

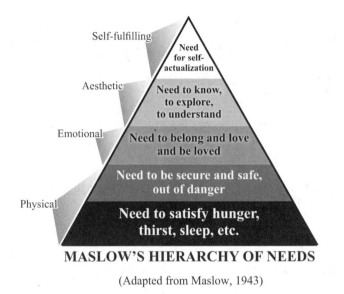

Self-fulfilling

Need
for self-
actualization

Aesthetic

Need to know,
to explore,
to understand

Emotional

Need to belong and love
and be loved

Need to be secure and safe,
out of danger

Physical

Need to satisfy hunger,
thirst, sleep, etc.

MASLOW'S HIERARCHY OF NEEDS

(Adapted from Maslow, 1943)

explored the lack of meaning in the lives of many people in nursing homes.

The Eden Alternative philosophy arises from the central principle that loneliness, helplessness, and boredom account for the bulk of suffering among frail elders. Eden advocates argue that these "plagues of the human spirit" cause suffering and mortality in excess of the underlying disease processes, and they must be eliminated in order to create a life worth living for elders.

These concepts may be difficult to quantify, but they are not hard for the careful observer to identify, and they can often be voiced, even by people with significant dementia. Researchers are beginning to look into these domains, which have been largely ignored in the past. For example, a recent study of adults aged 50 to 68 found a significant correlation between subjective symptoms of loneliness and higher blood pressure readings (Hawkley, Masi, Berry, and Cacioppo, 2006).

At the center of most definitions of well-being is identity, or what Kitwood (1997) calls personhood, which he defines in the following terms:

> It is a standing or status that is bestowed upon one human being, by others, in the context of relationship and social being. It implies recognition, respect, and trust. (p. 8)

Therefore, personhood has both intrinsic and extrinsic components. It speaks to the sacredness of the human spirit, but it also requires the recognition of others to be complete. In addition, it is very closely tied to social roles and self-esteem. Archbishop Desmond Tutu (1999) described a Zulu expression in this way:

> [A] person is a person through other persons. It is not, "I think, therefore I am." It says rather: "I am human because I belong. I participate, I share." (p. 31)

The interpersonal aspect of well-being is summarized by Dawn Brooker (2007) with the acronym VIPS: *valuing* people with dementia, treating them as *individuals*, seeing the world from their *perspective*, and providing a supportive *social environment* that recognizes the central importance of relationship. This suggests that even though some aspects of well-being may no longer be attainable by people with advanced dementia on their own, they can be maintained by the social environment. For example, even if a person no longer remembers her name, the recognition of her identity by her care partners can help maintain her well-being.

If the institutional model erodes well-being, then clearly it has a similar effect on personhood. The institutional focus on diseases and deficits (rather than the whole person), the loss of caregiving and decision-making opportunities, and one's subsequent disempowerment serve to undermine each of the components of personhood described above.

People with dementia who continue to write and speak about their experience echo this loudly and clearly. Richard Taylor (2007) speaks of his ongoing need "to have my personhood recognized. Please understand. I am still here" (p. 149). Bryden (2005) agrees: "How about separating us from the illness in some way? How about remembering we are a person with progressive brain damage?" (p. 143).

In his seminal work, *Dementia Reconsidered: The Person Comes First*, Kitwood (1997, pp. 46–47) postulated that even among well-intentioned care partners, the institutional model creates a multitude of small interactions that erode the personhood of people with dementia. He outlined 17 specific interactions, which he grouped under the term *malignant social psychology*. These are worth reviewing here because they speak to the range of potentially harmful interactions that a person with dementia can encounter in a world that is already difficult to navigate.

Treachery—forms of deception to manipulate or force compliance.

Disempowerment—either not allowing people to do things of which they are capable or not helping them complete a task.

Infantilization—addressing a person in a patronizing or childlike manner.

Intimidation—overt or implied threats.

Labeling—using diagnoses to interpret behavior or determine interactions.

Stigmatization—treating a person like a lesser entity.

Outpacing—providing information too quickly to be processed, thus rendering a person incapable of completing tasks she might otherwise have accomplished.

Invalidation—not acknowledging that a person's perceptions may feel very real to her.

Banishment—physical or psychological exclusion of an individual.

Objectification—treating a person like an object or task to be completed.

Ignoring—talking over a person, excluding her from the conversation.

Imposition—forcing someone to do something against her desires.

Withholding—refusing to answer a need.

Accusation—blaming an individual for being incapable or misunderstanding a situation.

Disruption—sudden interruption of a person, which could disturb her ability to attend to her environment.

Mockery—humor at the expense of others.

Disparagement—giving messages that are damaging to one's self-esteem.

Some of these are fairly obvious, but others, like outpacing, speak to a dynamic that even many seasoned professionals may not have noticed before. Outpacing can occur when a staff member gives information without allowing a person adequate time to process and respond. It can also occur when several people give simultaneous instructions to a person with dementia, a commonly observed sight. (As we will see, the best approach to a person with agitation involves only one person using slow, gentle conversation.)

Some of the foregoing interactions may sound rather cruel, but they are often played out in subtle ways that barely raise an eyebrow in the institution, or even in one's own home. Imposition, for example, does not have to be a full-scale assault. It can be as simple as giving a shower to someone who is protesting or resisting.

A closer look at Kitwood's list gives us further insight into the genesis of many behavioral expressions of dementia. These various interactions may actually cause such expressions or worsen preexisting ones. They may also impede communication, erode self-esteem, and force care partners to misinterpret people's words and actions.

This last effect has great importance in reframing our approach to behavioral expressions of dementia. Because of the way we view people with dementia, we are biased in the ways in which we hear their words and see their actions. Kitwood called this *positioning*. We often position the person with dementia as being less capable and less understanding than she really is. The effects of positioning are widespread in traditional care environments, and even nursing homes that are transforming their model of care struggle with this. Positioning can lead to the inability to recognize unmet needs, overdiagnosis of delirium or delusions, improper interpretation of words or actions, and exclusion of the person from the opportunity to engage in all aspects of meaningful life.

It should be mentioned that positioning and malignant social psychology are not confined to people with dementia. They can be devastating to all people who are physically frail or functionally dependent. All one has to do is sit in on a meeting where care professionals and family members discuss an elder in the third person, as if she isn't even in the room. Indeed, in many cases, she may not even have been invited to the meeting!

Now let's look once again at Maslow's hierarchy in the context of the work done by Carboni, Thomas, and Kitwood. It is clear that the institutional approach to care fails elders on all levels of the pyramid, and the chances for meaningful life and well-being are slim to none, particularly for those with dementia.

When I give presentations to physicians and clinical care staff, I often engage them in the following visualization exercise, compiled by Yvette Fuerderer.

A Day in Her Life
Close Your Eyes.
   Now imagine this being a typical day in your life:

You awake to the sound of loud voices and carts moving in the hallway outside your door. You want to keep sleeping, but someone has entered your room and thrown on the lights. It's someone you do not recognize. Your covers are drawn back and you feel cold and exposed. Your bottom garments are removed and then you are lifted out of bed and transferred into a wheelchair.

You are pushed down the bright and noisy hallway. Linen bins line the walls and the pungent smell of feces and urine stings your nostrils. You arrive in a bright room where your remaining clothing is removed and you are transferred onto a plastic bench. A shower is turned on. The temperature is not to your liking, but you are unable to verbalize that.

You are spoken to in short, "friendly" commands: "lift your arm," "hold on," "close your eyes," etc. You are methodically scrubbed with institutional-smelling soap, quickly rinsed, and then transferred back into the wheelchair. A small coarse towel is wrapped around you (you vaguely remember the large plush towels you had at home) and another is laid across your lap. You feel cold and exposed again.

Then you are wheeled through the same hallway. People are bustling about and nobody seems to notice or understand what you might be feeling. You hear things such as "Did you see the mess Mr. Jones made last night? Ugh!" and "When was Mrs. Hall's last BM?" and "Has anyone changed Bed 3 yet?"

Back in your room, you are dressed in an outfit someone else has chosen for you and placed in front of your TV (which is tuned to a station you never would have chosen for yourself). Breakfast is served on a plastic tray with plastic utensils. Even the food tastes plastic. Perhaps it wouldn't be so bad if it weren't cold again.

You are wearing a bib and drinking beverages from a Styrofoam cup. Before you have had time to finish one mouthful, another is fast approaching. Everyone is on a schedule. It's hard to believe that you'll never have another cheese omelet prepared "just for you," or coffee from one of your favorite cups. Fresh fruit? Just another thing of the past. Mid-meal, your attendant is called away. Eventually another appears and finishes the job . . .

Your bed needs changing, and since you are "in the way" you are moved into the hallway in front of the nurses' station along with some other residents. Periodically buzzers go off and calls go unanswered. You spend the rest of your morning gazing at the wall tiles. You're bored, lonely, and depressed. You wish you had some small bit of control in your life, but you've none.

You wonder where your family is. You desperately long for home. People assume that because you've shut down, your memory and mind have too, but you know where you are, and you know very well where you've been.

Workers come and go, but no one takes the time to stop and speak to you beyond "Hello." Minutes pass like hours, and you measure time by the arrival of your meals.

After lunch you have a BM and you're sitting in it. Won't anyone notice? . . . You know that only death will end your suffering.

When someone else decides it is time, you are brought back to your room. Dinner is ground up "something," you don't know what. (They've taken to grinding your food because it takes so long for you to chew.) Half the time you clamp your mouth shut because they're feeding you something you would never have let past your own lips when you were in control of your life. They settle for getting a cup of Ensure in you.

Again, when someone else decides it is time, you are changed for bed. You really don't mind though. Sleep is the only peace you know. You're given some applesauce that is gritty and tastes awful, and you are encouraged (before being forced) to accept it. These are your meds, and because your teeth have already been taken out for soaking, you are left with that flavor in your mouth for the rest of the night.

You close your eyes and pray for sleep, but it's a long time coming because your roommate is crying, like she does every night, that she wants to go home. You wish that someone would comfort her (or you). You wish that someone would lie down alongside you and stroke your hair until you fell asleep.

You have just imagined one day in the life of a resident living in a conventional nursing facility. Now imagine that this was going to be how you, or your loved ones, were going to live out *each day for the rest of your life.*

Admittedly, this story sounds pretty bleak. I inform my audiences that this story is true, based on Fuerderer's observations of how a woman's life changed after she moved into a conventional nursing home. Most listeners agree that even if they don't see all of these interactions every day, they all occur to some extent in even the best homes. I also reemphasize that the people who work in nursing homes are good, caring people stuck in a broken system that puts tasks ahead of relationships.

Then I close with one question: "Which psychotropic medication could you prescribe that would improve this woman's life?" No one has been able to answer that one yet.

This is a final flaw in medical treatment of behavioral expressions: medication is unlikely to help symptoms that are caused or perpetuated by a hostile environment. Make no mistake—the institution is an environment that is toxic to frail elders.

The institutional model is also toxic to those who work there. The employees of these nursing homes also suffer from plagues, which can be described as isolation, helplessness, and burnout (Horton, 2005). Isolation results from a model that compartmentalizes jobs and favors tasks over interpersonal interactions. Helplessness reflects a lack of autonomy similar to that experienced by elders, because the top-down hierarchy and the regulatory system also position *employees* as being less capable than they are. Burnout stems from the staff's tireless efforts to provide compassionate care within a system that does not value this quality.

Indeed, the lives of the direct care staff are equally vulnerable to what McLean (2007) calls the "cult of clock time and task." The model of care is so deeply institutionalized that it is built around the notion of clock time, rather than lived time—time that flows naturally, without following a predetermined schedule. The employees' (and elders') days are therefore divided according to work shifts, into a series of tasks to be done. These tasks are completely arbitrary when compared with the flow of a natural life; instead, they are designed around staffing hours. This causes an inevitable conflict when the flow of life does not conform, as is the case in people with or without dementia:

> Clock time imposes a uniformity and management over natural lived time by dividing it into standard measurable units. . . . Clock time transforms the self as lived into a compartmentalized collection of functions, similar to the items on the [Minimum Data Set] assessments or [Activities of Daily Living] task list that NAs check off as they proceed on their timely rounds. Thus it fragments the naturally lived time both of caregivers and care receivers, fracturing the inclination for intimacy that this relation brings. (McLean, 2007, p. 367)

McLean quotes Phillips (2001), who sees the damage on both sides, as the process "devalues both the actions of those identified as caregivers and strips those who would be seen as care recipients of much of their individuality and humanity" (p. 164).

Abandon hope, all ye who enter here.

Now, with a newfound understanding of our current flawed model of care, it is almost time to start building a new one. But first, one question remains: How do we explain the difficulties experienced by people with dementia who live *outside* of the nursing home?

Dementia in the Community:
When the Home Becomes an Institution

After all we have discussed, it is little wonder that people avoid nursing homes for as long as possible. What could ever be as good as living in your own home? Unfortunately, dementia changes one's experience of home, and the care environment is usually maladaptive to this process. For several reasons, staying home longer often worsens the situation and may actually lead to overmedication and more rapid decline.

According to the Alzheimer's Association (2009), over 70% of people with dementia in the United States live at home. Nearly 75% of the care provided to these people is unpaid care from relatives or friends.

A person with dementia in the community usually lives with a family member—either a spouse or sibling (who may be frail and have his or her own medical illnesses) or with a son or daughter (who may also have a job and/or child care responsibilities). This family member may not have the education and support necessary to understand and meet the needs of someone with dementia. In addition, most hired care is very expensive and not covered by insurance.

The person's care needs require a good deal of energy from family members, and the flexibility required to create a varied and sponta-neous environment is usually absent. At home, as in the nursing home, the focus is that dementia is a disease, and care of the body takes prece-dence. As home care becomes centered on task-doing, engagement and meaning are often lost.

As dementia progresses, many changes occur that may not be well managed in the home environment. There can be changes in the sleep–wake cycle, resulting in nighttime awakenings and walking around at odd hours. This puts further stress on the relative, who soon suffers the results of many nights of interrupted sleep. This is a major reason why people with dementia who live at home are given sedating medications. Unfortunately, these sleep–wake changes are not usually correctable with medication, and the result is often a further clouding of the senses or an unsteady gait. The resulting cognitive and func-tional decline often leads to a fracture, infection, or other event that can hasten nursing home placement.

Dementia can also cause losses of *initiation* and *executive function*. People become less able to initiate simple activities on their own, or to attend to tasks without frequent cueing. *Executive function* refers to basic problem-solving skills that may be impaired. There is a need for more structure, and when forced to be too self-reliant, the person with dementia can develop anxiety. A lone care partner cannot usually provide these supportive functions day and night. Even in assisted living facilities, people with dementia are too often left to their own devices, and without adequate cueing they can become restless and anxious, leading to more medication.

In 2008, I reviewed the records of all of the people who had moved to St. John's Home from the community over the previous 12 months. Virtually everyone had had a Folstein Mini-Mental State Exam as part of their evaluation in the first few weeks at our home. I correlated these results with the medications taken at home before the event that led to their move. I found that most people with mild to moderate dementia had been taking little or no antipsychotic medication at home. However, among those with more severe dementia, as measured by a Folstein score of 10 or less, 50% had been taking antipsychotic drugs at home. This shows that in the home environment, as in the nursing home, the use of sedating medication is a common response to advancing dementia.

A person with dementia tends to become isolated in the home. He can no longer participate in many previous social activities, and a caregiver may feel the need to separate him from much of the larger community. This social isolation can also further his decline.

Social Capital

Recent studies have shown the important effects of social connection and engagement on many aspects of health and well-being. There is a rapidly expanding literature on the importance of *social capital*.

> The new currency won't be intellectual capital. It will be social capital—the collective value of whom we know and what we'll do for each other. When social connections are strong and numerous, there is more trust, reciprocity, information flow, collective action, happiness, and, by the way, greater wealth. (Kouzes, 2000)

There are a number of emerging studies that correlate positive health outcomes with increased social capital. Pollack and von dem Knese-beck (2004) studied individual social capital in the United States and Germany, measured as the degree of participation in the community, reciprocity, and civic trust. They found that a low amount of social capital correlated with lower self-reports of health, more depression, and more functional limitations. Nilsson, Rana, and Kabir (2006) looked at social capital among 1,135 older adults in rural Bangladesh and found that low social capital was a significant predictor of poor quality of life. (It appears that this concept holds across cultures and socioeconomic strata.)

A three-year study of over 1,200 older adults in Sweden found that those with few or no social ties had a 60% increase in the risk of developing dementia (Fratiglioni, Wang, Ericsson, Maytan, and Winblad, 2000). A recently published Harvard study showed that increased social interaction slows memory loss in healthy older adults (Ertel, Glymour, and Berkman, 2008).

These studies suggest that if the home is a place where a person with dementia becomes isolated and disengaged from his social network, this can in turn worsen his overall health and well-being and even speed his cognitive decline.

Ironically, those things that give us meaning and fulfillment in our own homes can also be lost to the person with dementia. The very household that gave him his greatest pleasure may truly become an institution when it is no longer able to recognize and adapt to his individual needs and changing worldview.

Positioning in the Home

Because society has the same views of aging and infirmity that are seen in nursing homes, family members also employ positioning and malignant social psychology in their interactions with their loved ones. As in the nursing home, such disempowerment can have dire consequences. In his book *The Experience of Alzheimer's Disease: Life Through a Tangled Veil* (2001), psychologist Steven Sabat told two particularly memorable stories of positioning by family members.

> At the day center she attended, "Mrs. D." was considered "The Life of the Party." Born into a show business family, she was gregarious and witty, even though she had significant problems with memory, orientation, and visual-spatial tasks, and her Folstein Mini-Mental State Exam score was only 7/30, indicating severe dementia. She facilitated activities, led sing-alongs, and helped new members integrate into the group.
>
> At home, however, her husband described her to be sullen and quiet, and he had assumed most of her household chores because of her dementia. Mr. D. often spoke for his wife and he

would chide her whenever she made mistakes. He considered her incapable, due to her disease, and interpreted many of her comments as signs of her illness.

When Mrs. D. showed impatience in the morning because she had to "go to work," her husband assumed she was delusional. Mr. D. had positioned his wife as totally dependent and removed all opportunities for her to serve a useful role in the home, so she shut down.

When Dr. Sabat asked her directly about her "going to work," she answered very clearly that many of the people at the day center needed cheering up, and she saw this as a role she could fulfill:

> "Some of them are in bad shape, you know, that they couldn't remember a thing. I would try to help them. . . . I think it's a nice thing to do. Instead of me sitting down with the little I have . . . as things went by I would work, you know, with somebody just to keep them happy." (p. 128)

This is a good example of the social aspect of personhood, which defines the self in terms of how one fulfills a societal role. There was no such role for Mrs. D. at home, until her husband could be given the education to help him frame her condition in a more positive light and cultivate her strengths.

The story of Mrs. D. also illustrates that even though many people with advancing dementia have difficulty with verbal expression, they can make themselves understood with a listener who is perceptive and actively engages them to facilitate communication.

> "Mrs. R." had a similar degree of cognitive loss, and a caring husband who was even more overprotective than Mr. D. He would usually choose his wife's outfits, cut her food for her, and apply her makeup, even though she was able to do these tasks. He commented that she often "wandered aimlessly," which in fact was her response to being excluded from household activities. Her husband had assumed that she could not follow directions, so he did all the chores himself.
>
> As with Mrs. D., a totally different pattern emerged when Mrs. R. was at the day center. She was interactive and helpful with a variety of chores, such as arranging chairs, showing others to the rest room, and providing comfort and consolation to people in distress.

Brody (1971) wrote of a phenomenon she termed *excess disability*, which refers to a limitation that is greater than one's condition would dictate, as a result of environmental restrictions. The foregoing stories illustrate excess disability as a result of positioning and several types of depersonalizing interactions (malignant social psychology). It is clear that disempowering interactions are not limited to institutions.

But there is an even greater irony to our efforts to keep a loved one home as long as possible and avoid nursing home placement. The majority of nursing home admissions occur directly after an acute hospitalization, when it is determined that the individual can no longer safely return home. In other words, most people come to nursing homes only after a medical crisis necessitates their move. The result is that *most people are forced to make this major life transition when they are least able, physically and emotionally, to deal with it.*

A move to a nursing home is difficult enough. Now add the effects of a major illness, such as a stroke, hip fracture, or pneumonia, and the weakness and deconditioning that affect many elders after an acute illness. Delirium is often associated with a hospital stay, and people with dementia are likely to have worsening confusion in the hospital. Wouldn't it be nice if a nursing home was an option one would choose *before* the crisis occurred? I think it is clear why most people do not choose that option today, given the drawbacks already outlined.

In summary, institutional living is harmful to just about everyone, but even one's own home may fall far short of what the person with dementia needs for life fulfillment. How, then, do we best help people with dementia to live, or even thrive?

Three options seem most viable—change the home environment, change the nursing home environment, or create a new living environment that combines the best parts of both.

We have spent some time reviewing the shortcomings of the current approach to dementia, shortcomings that occur across all living environments. It is time to create a new paradigm. The next section will introduce an *experiential* model of care for people who live with dementia.

The text then outlines the components of this new model by looking at the promise of transformed nursing homes, because many people with dementia will continue to require care outside their own home. Then I will discuss the *aging in place* movement and its drawbacks, and suggest a new alternative that is taking hold even as I write these words.

PART 2

Shifts

CHAPTER 5

"Other Eyes"

Introducing the Experiential Model

THE FIRST PART OF THIS BOOK summarized the shortcomings of our current approach to dementia. Now it is time to construct a new model, engaging those "other eyes" and "other universes" that Proust (1929) described.

The biomedical model sees dementia mostly as neuropathology. However, viewing only what can be easily observed and measured is inadequate to our needs.

Levitin (2006) reminds us that sound waves have no particular pitch, tone, or beauty by themselves. It is only the way in which we hear and process those sounds that creates the experience of music. Applying his ideas to dementia, one can say that the physical and chemical changes that occur in the brain are of no consequence until they are *experienced* by the person with the changing brain.

That experience is more than simple structural and chemical defects; many other factors come into play, such as life history, relationships, values, interactions, and coping styles. Seeing dementia as a life experience and viewing the world through those eyes is the key to better understanding the needs of people with dementia.

It helps to compare and contrast the features of the biomedical

The Biomedical and Experiential Models of Dementia

	Biomedical Model	Experiential Model
Dementia defined	Progressive, irreversible, fatal	Shift in perception of world
Brain function	Loss of neurons and cognition	Brain is plastic, learning can occur
View of dementia	Tragic, costly, burdensome	Continued potential for life and growth
Research goals	Almost entirely focused on prevention and cure	Find ways to improve lives of those with dementia
Environmental goals	Protection, isolation, disempowerment	Maintain well-being and autonomy
Environmental attributes	Disease-specific living areas	Individualized, person-directed care
Focus of care	Programmed activities; Tasks and treatments; Less attention to care environment	Diverse engagement; Relationships; Care environment is critical
Staff/family role	"Caregiver"	"Care partner"
View of behavior	Confused, purposeless; Driven by disease and neurochemistry	Attempts to cope, problem solve, and communicate needs
Response to behavior	"Problem" to be "managed"; Medication, restraint	Care environment is inadequate; Conform environment to person
Behavioral goals	"Normalize" behavior; Meet needs of staff and families	Satisfy unmet needs; Focus on individual perspective
Nonpharmacologic approaches	Focus on discrete interventions	Focus on transforming care environment
Overall result	High use of meds; Continued suffering; Decreased well-being	Rare use of meds; Attention to spiritual needs; Improved well-being

model and an experiential model (also summarized in the table above). The biomedical model sees dementia as an irreversible, progressive, and ultimately fatal disease. The experiential model sees dementia as a shift in the person's perception of his or her world. The brain, while altered, remains somewhat plastic and is intimately tied to the surrounding environment. In fact, in many cases, individuals with dementia are more exquisitely sensitive to the attributes of their surroundings than the rest of us tend to be.

While the biomedical model views the disease process as one of loss of neurons and their associated cognitive functions, the experiential model holds that new learning can occur. (This happens all the time but is usually not recognized for its potential.)

The biomedical view sees dementia as tragic and costly. The predominant aim of research is to find a cure. The experiential view sees dementia as a challenge to make meaningful connections and improve the lives of all who live with the condition. This view doesn't put the lives of millions on hold while waiting for that elusive cure.

The biomedical view sees people with dementia as a burden and creates care environments that foster dependence. Biomedical dementia requires *caregivers*. The experiential view sees people for the gifts and abilities they continue to express to others. Experiential dementia creates *care partnerships* that empower all and maximize interdependence.

Several other attitudes and practices arise from the way we view dementia. The biomedical view leads us to conclude that people with dementia need a protective environment. This translates to isolation, disempowerment, and often institutionalization and overmedication. Furthermore, people's abilities are judged mainly through standardized cognitive tests, with broad conclusions drawn based on the resultant scores. Care planning and living environments are defined by the illness, not the individual.

McLean (2007) describes this process as follows:

> This model directs its attention to these finite processes and *away from the person who is experiencing them*. Thus, the subjective self is reduced to a mechanical object—the brain. In dementia in particular, when the brain as object does not properly function, it becomes devalued. (p. 368)

By contrast, the experiential model holds that well-being is not a function of cognitive skills, and that people may retain complex and integrative abilities far into their lives with dementia. People with dementia always remain unique individuals, and this uniqueness should be the driving force in their lives and their care. Autonomy should be preserved as far as possible.

The biomedical model focuses on tasks and treatments and pays relatively little attention to the many subtle interactions and features of the care environment. The experiential model focuses on relationships and sees interpersonal interaction and the overall environment as critical to the well-being of the person with dementia.

Each model also holds important implications for how we view and respond to behavioral expressions in people with dementia. The biomedical view sees such expressions as confused, purposeless, and neurochemically mediated. They are viewed as a "problem" that rests with the individual with the "disease" and that must be "managed." The primary goal is to return people to a "normal" state, often using psychotropic medication.

Kitwood (1997) remarked that "It has become far too easy to ignore the suffering of a fellow human being, and see instead a merely biological problem, to be solved by some kind of technical intervention" (pp. 43–44).

As a person who has lived with Alzheimer's disease, Taylor (2007) takes the challenge even further:

> The professionals become cheerleaders for caregivers, and sympathetic observers of me. The professionals are well-intentioned, but it is quicker and easier to "fix" caregivers than it is to listen to, understand, or even attempt to "fix" me. Caregivers' needs are clearer, more consistent and easier to address than mine! . . .
>
> Why not see us as a source of answers to our problems, rather than as a source of problems to which our caregivers need answers. (p. 67)

Thus the biomedical model centers on the perceptions and needs of the families and care staff, while discounting the unique perspective of the person who actually experiences the illness. This attitude leads one to position the opinions of the person with dementia as less valid and to resort to medication to "fix" the problem from the caregivers' perspective.

But if unmet needs are present, as studies show they usually are, then we must agree with Cohen-Mansfield's contention that "even if there was a 'magic pill' that stopped the agitated behavior occurring immediately and had no side effects, we shouldn't give it or start there" (2005, May). Why? Because doing so would still ignore those unmet needs and continue to rob the person of well-being.

The experiential model views people with dementia through their own eyes as far as possible. It views behavioral expressions as attempts to problem solve, cope with stressors, achieve control, or communicate needs. These expressions are viewed as *our* problem, because we have not provided the optimal environment for the person's well-being. The primary goal is to conform the care environment to the individual's needs, rather than to try to "normalize" the individual.

Pearce (2007) states:

> The path for encouraging the person with dementia to participate in
> life and human interactions lies in *our* opening to enter *her* world.
> When we are able to join the person in her world, we can see the
> many ways she continues to express her wisdom. (p. xvi)

In the biomedical model, nonpharmacological approaches tend to center on discrete interventions, such as a hand massage, washcloth folding, or pet therapy, with little attention to the overall environment. The caregivers (as they are called in the biomedical model) respond to a person's expressions of need by saying, "He's confused, because he has dementia."

While nonpharmacological approaches are a mainstay of the experiential model, the primary goal should be to *transform the care environment* (which we will discuss in detail in Chapter 6). In this model *care partners* (as I have come to call them) respond to such expressions of need by saying, "*I'm* confused, because I don't understand what he's trying to tell me."

As you can see, there are fundamental differences between the two views, and each leads to its own set of attitudes and approaches that create a stark contrast between the ways in which we might care for a person with dementia. This explains why one approach leans heavily on potentially harmful medications while the other almost eliminates their use.

A similar experiential approach to schizophrenia was suggested decades ago by the psychiatrist R. D. Laing (1965), who recommended a view he called existential phenomenology, which is the practice of discovering the other person's world and how he or she views it.

Laing also derided the fact that the biomedical approach places a higher value on objective data than subjective, because what can be measured objectively gives a limited view of each individual's experience. Sabat (2001) agrees: "No battery of standard objective neuropsychological tests . . . can open the door to the AD sufferer's interpersonal, social world and to the reality of the afflicted person's psychological experience in that world" (p. 315).

Kitwood (1997) remarked that "one of the most encouraging signs in recent years is that at last people with dementia are being recognized as having true subjectivity" (p. 70). This recognition is central to an experiential view of dementia.

These ideas suggest that an experiential model provides a "theory of relativity," in contrast to the "quantum" biomedical approach to dementia.

Before proceeding, I would like to comment on the use of language, both in this book and in the care of people with dementia. Transformational pathways stress the importance of looking critically at the language we use and conforming it to our new model of care.

This is not to disparage the hard work we have done in years past; rather, we understand that it can be difficult to engage a new paradigm if we use terminology that pulls us back into the old way of thinking.

Abraham Lincoln, in his 1862 address to Congress, said of the Civil War:

> The dogmas of the quiet past are inadequate to the stormy present.
> . . . As our case is new, so we must think anew and act anew. We must
> disenthrall ourselves, and then we shall save our country.

We need no less of a spirit of "disenthralling ourselves" from the past in order to "save" the care of people with dementia. So as we start to "think anew and act anew," we must heed the Eden Alternative's warning that "words make worlds."

To this end, I have attempted to meet the reader on some middle ground linguistically, then to slowly introduce new words to help us shift our paradigm. If the biomedical model is inadequate, then terminology rooted in the biomedical view of dementia must be replaced with words that reflect a person-directed, experiential view.

A prime example of this linguistic shift is my avoidance of the term *behavior problem*, which implies that the problem lies solely with the person with dementia. As this book amply demonstrates, a larger view is necessary to encompass the reality of the person in distress and to acknowledge the shortcomings of the care environment. I have now moved to the term *behavioral expressions*, because using the word *symptoms* puts us squarely in the realm of disease.

However, even the word *behavior* conjures up negative images, as our society uses the word so frequently to describe undesirable patterns of expression that must be "managed" or "controlled." My own language choices continue to evolve, but my best substitute at present is *expressions of need*.

Another personal shift has been my use of the term *care partner*. The intent is to replace the word *caregiver*, which suggests that care is a one-way street and the person with dementia is incapable of reciprocating in any way.

The term *care partner* is central to the philosophy of Eden at Home (created by Laura Beck—see Resources), which applies the principles of the Eden Alternative to home- and community-based care. In this case, the tendency for community care to become institutionalized is counteracted by the creation of care partnering teams, in which the person with the identified care needs is an active participant.

I first came across this concept after reading a wonderful description by Bryden (2005):

> Adopting a sole identity as our care-giver highlights our illness and strips both of us of other identities; we have become care-giver and sufferer, in a relationship of co-dependence. . . .
>
> In this role, you may soon feel overwhelmed by the multitude of tasks, of remembering for two, of planning and organizing for two, of covering up our deficits, and grieving over our losses, rather than looking for what remains. You can quickly become exhausted, sad, depressed and in despair. . . .
>
> At the same time, if we adapt a sole identity as a sufferer of our illness, we learn helplessness. We lose more function, and show an excess disability. . . . This will only add to your burdens as a care-giver, and exacerbate the problem for both of us. . . .
>
> We need to move away from labeling ourselves as care-giver and sufferer, towards becoming a care-partnership, in which we accept, collaborate, and adapt to new roles within the journey of dementia. . . . In this care-partnership, the person with dementia is at the center of the relationship, not alone as an object to be looked at, as merely a care recipient. Instead, we become an active partner in a circle of care. (pp. 149–150)

Language choices are also incredibly important in our interpersonal interactions, not only when talking to people with dementia, as we will explore in detail, but in communicating with other care partners. The words we choose communicate powerful messages that can potentially "poison" other interactions.

Here is an example I often pose to care staff: Let's suppose that Mrs. Jones decides not to take her bedtime dose of medication. Perhaps she has an upset stomach, or maybe she had fallen asleep and didn't appreciate being awoken to swallow more pills. In typical fashion, it is documented that "Resident *refused* her evening meds." If you were a staff member covering the floor and you did not know Mrs. Jones, what would you think when you read that entry?

I have posed this scenario to audiences across the United States and halfway around the world, and the answer is always the same: "It sounds like she's difficult, disagreeable, combative, or a troublemaker. I would go into her room expecting an argument."

Note how the simple word *refused* has poisoned the attitude of all who will be approaching Mrs. Jones! This use of loaded words is ubiquitous, even in the best medical care settings. It is intimately involved in our tendency to "position" people with dementia.

As Richard Taylor (2007) tells us, there can be much more to the refusal of medication than meets the eye:

> I suspect that not taking my meds is my way of saying "NO" to the disease. It is my way of remaining in control of me. . . .
>
> The longer I live with Alzheimer's disease, the less important the pills become to me. The farther along I am in the disease, the more important the pills become to my caregivers. I want them to understand that I don't want to swallow a bitter pill twice a day—nor do I want to be the bitter pill that my caregivers must swallow each day. (p. 200)

Thus a look into the *experience* of Alzheimer's disease gives us insights we would never have found in the biomedical approach.

Eden Alternative board member Sarah Rowan told me the story of her husband, Joseph, who lived with Alzheimer's disease. She recalled a picnic they had one day, when he dug up a small sapling to free it from encroaching rocks and presented it to her as a gift:

> I smiled at him and said, "Oh, Joseph, what makes you the miracle you are?" He looked at me and said back to me, "What makes you the miracle you are?"
>
> I thought about how it felt hearing my own words repeated back, and I thought, "If every word I spoke were echoed back to me, would I feel celebrated, or just tolerated?"
>
> . . . Words can be a tool of torture or an instrument of inspiration. The words we choose can determine if a situation will be escalated or de-escalated and if a person will be humanized or de-humanized.

Our choice of words also has a powerful effect on how we interpret specific expressions of need. Subsequent chapters will apply this concept to such terminology as *wandering, combativeness, delusions, paranoia,* and *hallucinations.*

The following box displays a summary of the experiential model in the form of action steps (which will help guide our approach to care in the third part of the book).

The Experiential Model: Action Steps

- Each person with dementia has a unique life story and individual needs.

- Although there are cognitive deficits, many complex abilities are preserved, which should be identified and cultivated.

- The brain remains plastic, and new or compensatory learning can still occur.

- The primary task for enlightened care is to cultivate close relationships throughout the care environment.

- The manner in which we provide care can have profound effects on the individual's abilities and overall well-being.

- Well-being is not dependent on cognitive or functional ability and should be maximized in all people.

- People with dementia can be thought of as inhabiting a "parallel universe," existing in the same time and space as ours, but with somewhat different rules and values. We must strive to acknowledge and understand these universes and find a common ground for care.

- We must work hard to find unmet needs and adapt the care environment to meet those needs as far as is safe or practical.

- The world of the person with dementia changes over time, and so we must also change and adapt to their evolving needs.

- We must use creativity and collaboration to create a life worth living for people with dementia.

Because transformation of the care environment is such a central feature of the experiential approach, I will begin by describing what this entails. Chapter 6 will review the basic physical, operational, and interpersonal features of this transformed care environment.

Chapter 7 will expand upon this by examining some important areas that are often overlooked in the process of transformation. Then Chapter 8 will back up and look at the larger view of aging in society and present some challenging ideas about future directions in elder care and care for all those who will live with dementia in the 21st century.

The third part of the book will apply the experiential approach to a number of common scenarios to show how this philosophy can be put to practical use in our everyday interactions.

CHAPTER 6

Putting the
Dragon to Sleep

Deinstitutionalizing Care Environments

ANY COMPREHENSIVE PATHWAY to transform institutional care requires three components. Just as the institution, whether it is a nursing home or an individual's home, has physical, operational, and interpersonal features, the process of moving away from the institutional model requires change in all three of these areas. As with the earlier description of the institutional model, the interpersonal aspects of transformation are the least visible, but they are the most important in bringing about real change.

The Nursing Home

There are many sources available that outline the details of institutional transformation. The following comments are not meant to be exhaustive. The Resources includes many such sources. This section outlines some of the basic considerations that a home should review in its transformative journey and shows how these changes can be instrumental in caring for people with dementia.

We will start with transformation of the physical environment, because it is easiest to visualize. In practice, however, physical renovation should be the *last* step, not the first.

Physical Environment

The physical environment is important to the person with dementia because it is a major contributor to one's functional status, as well as to feelings of familiarity, comfort, and security. The physical environment includes several components: the size and layout, the decor and furnishings, and the lighting and acoustic environment as well.

When it comes to nursing homes and their living areas, bigger is definitely not better. A large scale is often more cost-effective, but it has several drawbacks for people who live in the home. The majority of Americans who live in houses, farms, or small apartments will find the traditional high-rise nursing home very daunting in terms of comfort and familiarity. Even city dwellers who are accustomed to high-rise living are used to having a private apartment, and traditional nursing homes leave little room for privacy or solitude.

From a functional standpoint, a person with decreased strength and endurance will find it difficult to walk long distances to get to a living room or dining area. Many people who come to nursing homes become more functionally disabled simply by virtue of these increased distances. Elders often walk more independently as a result of renovations that move them to smaller living environments.

As a general rule, the more people there are in a living area, the less likely any single person will be able to experience choice or individualized care. People are less likely to be well known to their care partners. The larger floor plan is harder for people with dementia to internalize. Large and crowded living areas also result in higher levels of background noise and commotion, both from the occupants and from the activities of the staff around them.

The first task in changing the physical environment, therefore, is to make it smaller. If renovations are not feasible, there are many ways to make the home *feel* smaller for those who live there. Familiarity and comfort can be improved by providing areas where a person can find solitude. Cohen and Day (1993) observe that most environments "do not provide sufficient variation in the levels of privacy available." They suggest that "a gradient from public to private spaces offers residents control over the desired level of sensory stimulation, social interaction, and involvement in activities" (p. 14).

While one's personal living space may not be easily enlarged, bringing as much individual meaning to the space at hand can increase attachment and engagement. Allowing personal furniture and meaningful artifacts is another good step.

Cohen and Day add that our institutional approach to care has destroyed the privacy and sanctity of the bedroom. "Also lost is a clear identification of [the bedroom's] function, which can prompt and support appropriate patterns of behavior" (p. 17). Therefore, it should come as no surprise that behavioral expressions that involve a loss of boundaries often have an origin in the way people are forced to live in nursing homes.

Look at the comfort of the living space from the elder's perspective. Are the bed and chair comfortable? How is the lighting? Is the decor warm and pleasing to the eye, or cold and institutional? How often is agitation or anxiety intertwined with physical discomfort?

Burger (1992) reported a woman in a nursing home who was constantly getting up at night and falling. Attention to the usual factors (such as bathroom needs, pain control, food, and drink) was unsuccessful in alleviating this nighttime pattern. Then an aide decided to experience the room from the elder's perspective. She lay down on the bed and was immediately struck by the glare of a light from the hallway that landed on her eyes. The light was extinguished, and so were the falls.

The Special Case of Lighting

The need for adequate light becomes increasingly important as we age. Several factors accompany aging of the eyes. There is a slower response to changes in light levels, and the pupils are generally smaller and let in less light. In addition, the lens becomes denser and begins to take on a yellowish hue. Add to this the possibility of cataracts, macular degeneration, or other eye disorders; the net effect is that much less light gets to the optic nerve to produce a clear visual image.

At age 65, we need about three times as much light as a young person; at 85, we need up to five times as much. Unfortunately, most living environments do not provide this. Increased attention to energy efficiency and budgetary concerns also contribute to inadequate lighting.

Most nursing homes fall far short of providing adequate light. A survey of over 50 nursing homes in four states showed inadequate light levels in 45% of all hallways, 51% of bedrooms, and 17% of activity areas (Sloane, Mitchell, Calkins, and Zimmerman, 2000). Another study of ambient light levels showed them to be at less than half of the *minimum* standard for these environments (Deremeik et al., 2007).

There are several reasons why this is so important. First, we need enough light to complete our normal activities of life (such as washing, dressing, and eating), as well as to engage in other enjoyable activities (such as reading or doing craftwork). Inadequate light is a major factor creating functional dependence and poor quality of life among older people (Chen, Sloane, and Dalton, 2003).

A second consideration is the need for regular doses of natural light. Natural light is a primary factor in running the body's "biological clock," setting the day–night tempo called the circadian rhythm. Without good doses of natural light, or light of similar wavelength and intensity, the body loses its cues for sleep and wakefulness.

The sleep patterns that change naturally with age are further exaggerated by this loss of circadian rhythm. Clapin-French (1986) showed that people with normal sleep quality who move into nursing homes develop significant problems. At least part of this is due to the disruption of the body clock. Add a component of dementia to this, and the result can be devastating. In fact, disruption of the circadian rhythm has been linked to worsening cognitive function and depression, so the problems are compounded. (Sunlight also increases levels of serotonin, one of our mood-enhancing brain chemicals.)

It should go without saying that poor lighting increases the risk of falls and fractures. Lack of natural light compounds the problem further by reducing vitamin D and bone production. A study of elders in Japan showed that those who had 15 minutes of sunlight on their faces and hands, on an average of 236 clear days per year, had 84% fewer fractures than a group who did not (Sato, Metoki, Iwamoto, and Satoh, 2003).

Proper attention to lighting addresses not only the quantity of light, but also the quality. Older eyes are more susceptible to glare, caused by improper light positioning or poorly chosen colors and materials used in flooring and other surfaces. State and federal standards for elder living environments are woefully inadequate. Also, most regulators and staff are younger adults who evaluate the lighting without remembering to look "through the elders' eyes."

In addition to causing glare, flooring can have a negative effect on the function of people with dementia when certain colors and patterns cause confusion with safe foot placement. Some people with dementia see certain color borders as a drop-off and won't step across. I have seen people who have great difficulty placing their feet on floors with certain design patterns, even though they are flat. In some cases, more ambient light can help; in others, the design needs to be changed.

How do we improve this critical factor of lighting in our living environments? First and foremost, we must recognize that needs should be dictated by the visual limitations of those who reside there, rather than our own abilities. When renovating, bring elders into the design process from the outset (more about this in the section on operational environment).

Next, think of four basic factors: ambient light, targeted light, glare, and natural light. Ambient (background) light should be indirect and reflected, rather than exposed bulbs that shine in one's eyes, causing glare in some areas and shadows in others. Targeted light should be positioned appropriately for the activities that will be taking place in a given area. Surfaces below eye level should absorb light instead of reflecting it up into the eyes. Floors, paving, walls, and furniture should be chosen with colors and surfaces that are easy to discern but don't cause undue glare. Daylight should be brought into the home whenever possible. Skylights and high clerestory windows can provide maximum sun illumination with less glare than light coming through low windows and doors. An excellent review of these principles can be found in a paper by Brawley and Noell-Waggoner (2008).

The Sound and the Fury

Another physical consideration whose contribution to distress is greatly underappreciated is the acoustic landscape of the nursing home. Here's a simple exercise that can be very enlightening:

> Next time you are in a nursing home or other care environment, sit down and close your eyes for a few moments. Relax, breathe slowly, and focus your thoughts on the sounds around you. What do you hear?
>
> If the home is still ensconced in the institutional model, you may hear overhead pages, intercoms, call bells, or chair alarms. Imagine how the sound of disembodied voices is experienced by a person who is disoriented. Note that the call bells and alarms are intended to be loud and somewhat annoying so that they are not ignored by staff. Imagine how a person with dementia feels when these sudden loud noises occur in her environment.
>
> Next, listen for other sounds that you would not find in the home environment—the "thud-thud" of the pill crusher, the elevator's arrival bell, and the constant sounds of the fax machine, copier, and phones at the nurses' station.
>
> Now, listen to the television in the lounge. What does it sound like? Are the commercials loud and jarring? Does the sound of

gunfire and screaming accompany a police drama? Do you hear the loud angry voices from a soap opera or a contentious talk show? We tend to let these sounds roll off us, but how do they feel to a person with dementia?

Finally, listen to the voices you hear around you. Start with the quantity and volume. Does it feel noisy and hectic around you? Listen to the tone of the voices. Do they sound relaxed or stressed? Does the atmosphere feel warm and inviting, or cold and harried? Imagine experiencing these sounds and moods day after day. Are you in a place where you could relax and feel at home? Doesn't it feel like a "battle zone" at times?

We will explore these latter concepts in greater detail later, when discussing the specifics of agitation. As mentioned earlier, there are many other trappings of the institution that are not found in anyone's home. Many culture change organizations can provide detailed advice on how to do away with nurses' stations, medication carts, overhead pages, or other institutional features.

Next, I will focus on the interpersonal environment, as this will dictate the operational changes that must be made in order to support the transformation of the nursing home.

Interpersonal Environment

The drawbacks of the institution are complex and pervasive, but they can be gradually dismantled by cultivating an environment whose interactions are similar to those that are found in one's home. There are several aspects that provide antidotes to the plagues of institutionalization.

First and foremost is the creation of close and continuing relationships among all members of the nursing home community. For better or worse, we know our family members well. We understand who they are, where they come from, what makes them tick. We know what displeases them and what brings them joy and fulfillment. Imagine how such knowledge could help us meet the needs of our elders with dementia.

One of the core values of the Pioneer Network (see Resources) is that "Relationship is the fundamental building block of a transformed culture." Like family members, the people in our care need to be well known to us—not simply as a list of diagnoses or a litany of functional abilities and disabilities, but as whole people. This has implications for staffing as well as for many routine nursing home procedures, such as the comprehensive care plan.

Next, it is important to find ways to restore choice and control to elders and those who are closest to them. This not only reaffirms the basic ethic of self-determination, it restores usefulness to elders by returning to them the ability to be part of the decisions that affect their lives and the lives of those around them. It creates collaboration among elders, families, and staff, rather than an us-versus-them mentality that erects barriers to care.

Restoring choice and control in people with dementia can be as simple as pointing to the food on a plate and asking, "What would you like to try first?" It may be as basic as being sure that each person attends his own care plan meeting and speaking directly to him, rather than talking about him as if he isn't in the room. It also requires that we open our minds to the fact that people with dementia may retain more insight than we often expect them to have.

It is also important to provide opportunities for elders to continue to be caregivers as well as care recipients. Most of our elders have lived through wars and economic booms and busts. They have raised children, pursued careers, and acted as mentors and advisers over the years. We have seen how the institutional nursing home fosters dependency and causes people to feel helpless and of little use to the world. As with decision making, people with dementia can almost always give care on some level, whether by reading to a child, watering a plant, stroking a cat—even "nurturing" a doll, as people with advanced dementia may do.

Dr. Vicki Rosebrook (2002), executive director of the Macklin Intergenerational Institute, studied the effect of an intergenerational program on the personal and social development of preschoolers who interacted regularly with people with dementia. She found that the children, upon reaching school age, were nearly 6 months ahead of their peers in several developmental markers. A follow-up study performed 4 years later (Rosebrook, 2007) showed them to be 11 months advanced. The greatest differences were seen in areas of cooperation, expressing their emotions, and social graces.

Rosebrook theorizes that the three Eden plagues of loneliness, helplessness, and boredom have counterparts in the needs of preschool children, namely interaction, guidance, and exploration. In this way, people with dementia can help provide what these children need and receive antidotes for the plagues of institutionalization at the same time. The study shows how wrong it is to assume that people with moderate degrees of dementia cannot guide and be role models for young children.

Another offshoot of close relationships is the ability to fill each elder's life with meaning. The better we know someone, the better we are able to choose conversation or activities that hold individual value, and the greater fulfillment we can bring to someone's life. This can begin with an investigation of each person's history, including family, career, hobbies, values, and spirituality.

It is also helpful to ask about a person's "simple pleasures" and how they might be re-created by the care environment. A simple pleasure is just what the name implies: a simple activity one engages in regularly that brings pleasure and satisfaction. Everyone has one or more of these. The key is that each person's simple pleasures are highly individualized and often carry special meaning for the person. In fulfilling a simple pleasure, it is critical to obtain all of the little details that make it a special experience. For example, a cup of coffee at sunrise may be a simple pleasure for many people, but each person will want the coffee prepared a certain way, perhaps served in a favorite mug. Care partners may well discover that many of these pleasures are not so "simple" to re-create in an institutional nursing home.

The simple pleasure is an important tool for creating experiences rich in being and individual meaning, and it also helps organizations learn to collaborate across departmental lines to bring these to fruition. This in turn provides a process for planning how larger activities can be organized in order to create meaningful rituals and decide how other important events are to be celebrated (see Chapter 7).

Finally, it is important to foster an environment that allows for spontaneity and variety. Many people complain that nursing homes need "more activities and more activities personnel." Scheduled events (such as movies, concerts, and bingo games) do provide enjoyment, but much of the joy in life is unplanned, flowing from personal relationships and from a diverse and lively environment. We need to be able to attend to our elders' needs as they occur, instead of simply waiting for the next scheduled activity.

These are the attributes of home—nurturing relationships with people you know well, choice and control over daily life, opportunities to give care, variety, spontaneity, and meaning in everyday life. This is the foundation of the transformed environment, and its impact on the care of people with dementia is enormous. (The next chapter will further explore activity and meaning.)

Among care staff, transformation needs to start with education about these basic concepts, long before any physical or operational changes are undertaken. These concepts cannot be legislated; they must be internalized by those within the network of care, starting with those who wish to lead the transformative process. Fox (2007) sums it up succinctly: "You grow first" (p. 55).

As I mentioned in Chapter 4, many of these interpersonal features are lacking in community settings as well as in the nursing home. The dragon can reside in our own homes, if we let it.

Operational Environment

The primary function of operational change is to better enable the development of those interpersonal interactions that characterize a nourishing environment. Therefore, as already summarized, our operations must enable the development of close and continuing relationships, increase choice and control over one's environment, create the ability to answer the needs of the moment, and restore variety, spontaneity, and meaning to life.

Relationships and Staffing

In order to strengthen relationships, several goals must be met. The first is to keep care partnerships as close and continuous as possible. This has huge implications for staffing. Agency personnel may be skilled and caring, but it is next to impossible for a person who rotates from one nursing home to another to understand the individual needs of the people in her care.

Like so many of these elder care concepts, this is especially critical in dealing with people who have dementia who may not be able to make their needs known clearly. It follows that use of agency staff is counterproductive to the goals of transformation. Eliminating agency staff is difficult work, given the national shortages of nurses and nursing assistants, but as our nursing home has shown, this can be accomplished with gratifying results:

> At St. John's Home in Rochester, New York, we were using hundreds of shifts of agency staff every month to help care for our 475 elders. Our total agency budget was over $3 million annually. As a result, we had many care issues and survey deficiencies in spite of a relatively low full-time staff turnover rate of 35%.
>
> In 2001, I took a leadership group to a retreat with Dr. William Thomas, founder of the Eden Alternative. We asked how we

could fold agency staff into the Eden model. His matter-of-fact reply: "You can't—you have to eliminate agency staff." This seemed next to impossible at the time, yet the decision of one local agency to significantly raise its fee spurred us to action.

Our CEO, administrator, and director of nursing met with all nurses and aides on all shifts over the next several weeks. They asked everyone what they liked about St. John's, what they didn't like, and what would make it the ideal place to work. Then they asked the agency staff who regularly worked here why they came to St. John's so often and what it would take for them to consider full-time employment here. Their responses led us to examine the needs of people who prefer part-time or agency work over full-time employment, such as child care and flexible hours. A date was set to begin eliminating agency staff, and those who wanted to continue their affiliation were given applications and encouraged to become St. John's Home employees. Those who chose to apply knew that their regular affiliation with our home had given us knowledge of their talents and abilities.

Many steps were taken to improve the work environment: we benchmarked with other homes to adjust our wages and pay differentials for evening and night shifts, increased our flexibility with work schedules, and built an on-campus child care center with preferred rates for employees. The interview and hiring processes were streamlined to be more user-friendly. New rules made it more difficult for supervisors to call in agency staff so that more energy could be directed toward finding other solutions to meeting our needs.

Many other initiatives were also undertaken over the next several months to help increase the "warmth" of the organizational environment and solicit input from all staff. New rituals—both to welcome new employees and to honor established ones—were introduced.

Over the next 18 months, our agency staffing dropped to zero, and we have now been agency-free for over 5 years. Our regulatory surveys have improved significantly, as have our satisfaction survey results. Most astounding is that our annual full-time staff turnover has fallen each year: in 2006 it was down to 14%, and in 2008 we were at just 8.6%!

A 2002 study by the American Health Care Association reported average annual staff nurse and director of nursing turnover rates of around 50% nationwide, and certified nursing assistant (CNA) turnover averaged 71%. Only two states had average CNA turnover rates of less than 40%. Nationally, even the turnover of nursing home administrators is several times higher than that of our overall staff.

We have now implemented permanent nurse and CNA assignments in each living area. With each of these changes, I see another quantum of success with nonpharmacological approaches as we strengthen relationships and create more meaning and connection for our elders.

Permanent assignment of staff can be a hard sell for many nurses and CNAs who are frustrated by particularly "difficult" elders or family members. However, those who have made the transition have found that the cultivation of closer relationships has had a positive effect on their interactions and their overall satisfaction. Being "in it for the long haul" helps develop our ability to see another person's point of view and increases the willingness of all parties to find collaborative, win–win solutions to conflict.

Permanent assignments are not just for the nursing department. It is not uncommon for doctors, social workers, or therapists to be permanently assigned, but how about members of the housekeeping or maintenance departments? Our environmental service staff has become quite invested in the elders who they have come to know through this system. Our maintenance workers have gotten to know the nursing staff and elders in a particular living area and are able to anticipate and prevent many physical and mechanical issues as a result of their close association with their adopted "neighborhoods."

We have members of the Business Office, Human Resources, and Buildings and Grounds departments who regularly facilitate activities for a given neighborhood. One of our dining service employees, Denise, regularly brings cookies to people with dementia living in her mother's neighborhood. She related that she hadn't thought many of the people recognized her, but when she returned from a week's vacation, Denise was surprised when several people with advanced dementia asked her where she had been and told her that they had missed her.

Care Planning

How else can the organization help our elders to become well known? One major area is that of care planning. Several things can be done to enhance this process. The most basic is to be sure the elder, family, and primary nurse and aide have every opportunity to be present and participate in the care plan. Care plans are best designed by the elder and those who know her best. It is staggering how often these people are not involved in many of the care planning decisions in most organizations.

Second, the care plan needs to be holistic. It needs to tell us each person's story, her important accomplishments, her relationships, and what is most meaningful to her. It should not just be a litany of diagnoses and functional descriptors.

There are two valuable tools that help us to reimagine the traditional care planning process. The first is the use of the *first-person narrative*. Writing the care plan in the first person gives a personal dimension to the care plan that brings each individual to life. Even for individuals who are unable to give their own account, writing the plan of care as if they are speaking for themselves brings a more holistic and person-directed dimension to the narrative.

The second concept is the *video care plan*. This is simply a slideshow in which the first-person narrative is combined with photos and images that imprint the uniqueness of the individual in the minds of those who watch. Use of a specially chosen musical accompaniment and pictures from earlier life can help to create this indelible image. The video can also serve as a remembrance of an elder's life after he passes away. Organizations such as It's Never 2 Late can provide software and support for this process (see Resources).

There are more ways to facilitate relationship building than can be described here, and many readers will come up with ideas unique to their own situations. Later, we will use these building blocks to drastically reshape the landscape of care approaches for people with dementia.

Empowered Work Teams

The operational key to restoring choice and control is the creation of neighborhood teams to address many of the day-to-day decisions in the home. After deepening relationships and moving to permanent assignments, teams can be created from small groups of elders, their primary care partners, and members of other departments of the home.

After a period of education (in which members learn the basics of team building, holding meetings, assigning roles, resolving conflict, and reaching consensus), it will become the function of these groups to decide how life will be lived in their neighborhood. This is the point where transformation and empowerment truly become manifest.

Horton (2005) offers this process as an antidote for her "three plagues of isolation, helplessness, and burnout" for staff (p. 179): (1) empathic leadership and relationship building provide the antidote to isolation; (2) sharing of knowledge and decision making combats helplessness; and (3) creating a culture of empowerment, education, emotional support, and creativity helps to prevent burnout.

Once again, this is a slow and incremental process that is more fully described by the specific literature of the various culture change movements. The result of this process is a "flattening" of the traditional top-down hierarchy that has long disempowered elders and hands-on care partners. Instead of the hierarchical organizational structure described earlier, we strive for an image that resembles an archery target, with the elders in the bull's eye, the place of highest importance, and the direct care staff in the innermost ring beside them.

With this new view of the organization, directors and managers can learn to enable the development of operational policies that are centered on the needs of the elders, and help the neighborhood teams to establish a true model of person-directed care. A new attitude is cultivated that, as managers, we actually work for those we manage, rather than for those who manage us. There are many books available that describe this philosophy of *servant leadership*. With this inversion of the hierarchy of service, the flow of accountability now points in the proper direction—toward the elder. Care-partnering opportunities increase when elders are involved in these decision-making processes. The incorporation of animals, plants, and children into the daily life of the home is another useful step in restoring elders' caring roles.

Once we have created meaningful relationships and have empowered elders and their care partners, we have the knowledge, teamwork, and motivation to further individualize care. Employees can be more cross-trained and become flexible enough to share in the life of the neighborhood, rather than being chained to a particular department or job description.

Of course, nurses may always dispense medications, and dieticians will always review meal choices; individuals will retain certain areas of expertise by virtue of their training and licensure. However, each person can also respond to the needs of the moment, thus contributing to the creation of meaning and joy in an elder's day—and do so with the support of coworkers and without fear of being criticized for goofing off or not staying on task. This increased flexibility of the living environment flows from the operational changes that empower each care partner to put the person before the task. Cohen-Mansfield and Bester (2006) reviewed the attributes of a home in Australia that improved care by creating a more flexible environment:

> The director of nursing summarized his philosophy about the role of staff members in the following way: "If, when I come into the unit in the morning, I see all the beds made, and the residents all dressed, I am concerned. But, if I see that not everything has been done, and

that staff members are eating breakfast and joking with the residents, I know everything is fine." (p. 541)

Keeping the Horse Before the Cart

It is best to delve deeply into interpersonal and operational changes before any major physical alterations are accomplished. A prime example is meal service. In order to move from the very traditional model of fixed mealtimes (with centralized food preparation and plastic trays) to a model of family-style dining (cooked locally and served at individually preferred times), a lot of operational and interpersonal work has to be accomplished. The same is true with live-in pets. Failed attempts at these changes often result from rushing through the interpersonal work to get to the more "visible" aspects of culture change.

For those still engulfed in the medical model, it can be difficult to envision how all of this can happen. It seems there aren't enough hours in the day and it sounds chaotic. It would be, doing our jobs as we do them in the current system. However, through slow, incremental organizational change, ongoing education, and encouragement of interpersonal growth, a true home for elders can be created. The secret lies in a strong commitment to transformation, embraced and modeled by the formal leadership of the organization. Many years ago, Gandhi challenged us to "become the change we wish to see."

It is possible to achieve some measure of success without all three components of change. However, like a three-legged stool, the most balanced homes have worked on all three aspects. Once again, interpersonal change remains the key. I have seen very institutional-looking homes that have achieved remarkable success in caring for people with dementia and reducing medications due to the extensive relationship work they have done.

On the flip side, there are many homes that rush to put the physical changes in place and short-change the interpersonal aspects of transformation. These always fall short of true enlightened care. I have seen many beautiful, newly built or renovated homes that nevertheless are cold environments. This is because the people who work there still have institutional hearts and minds.

As Malcolm Gladwell stated in *The Tipping Point* (2002), the influence of one's physical environment can be powerful. However, in caring for people with dementia, it still takes a back seat to interpersonal transformation—otherwise people who live at home would not have the behavioral expressions they often display, nor receive the amount of sedating medication they do. Clearly much more is needed than simply creating a homey physical environment.

Home and Community Living

If home- and community-based care have also been institutionalized, then the same three aspects of transformation must be examined as they apply to these environments. Here, the dragon is not always as obvious, but he may exert an equally harmful effect.

From a physical standpoint, the home needs to continue to serve the needs of the person with dementia. Many obvious aspects come to mind, such as removing obstacles to walking, using lock-out switches on stoves and other appliances, and engaging the available technology that helps people to maintain their independence in this setting. Careful attention should be paid to issues of light and sound, as these are often suboptimal in the home as well.

In order for the home to adapt to the changing perceptions of the person with dementia, the family may need to make changes that do not always make sense on the surface. For example, if an object in the house begins to bother the person for some reason (such as a photo or a piece of furniture that triggers an unpleasant memory), it may be the best solution to simply remove it from the environment so that it does not continue to be a source of irritation.

The same interpersonal considerations apply regardless of the living environment. First, relationships should be as close and continuous as possible. Rapidly changing home health aides can be just as disruptive as changing staff in the nursing home. Second, autonomy should be preserved as far as possible. As we have seen, it is far too easy for families to take over all aspects of care, leaving the person with dementia feeling useless. Part of this involves finding ways for the person to continue to provide care to others, by helping maintain the house, caring for a pet or plants, and having input into how each day is structured.

As with the nursing home, we must be sure that the care needs of the person with dementia do not force the home environment to lose all spontaneity and variety. Daily activities need to continue to hold meaning and connection for the person whose cognition and needs will evolve over time. It is important for families to remember that, although a particular activity is something a person "always liked to do," this may change as dementia changes the person's perceptions and abilities. The inability of family members to adapt to such patterns of change often causes the distress that leads to sedating medications.

Operational transformation of the home is very tricky because the environment needs to provide increasing structure and guidance while preserving a degree of control and autonomy for the person with dementia. This is one of the most difficult concepts to bring to community life. In the community, care partners tend to usurp the autonomy of the person with dementia. When care partners are challenged to allow more choice, there are two common responses: (1) "Allowing him to choose is too risky," or (2) "I have tried, but he does not seem able to make those decisions."

The same barriers often occur when managers are trying to empower their staff in institutions. In both cases, this relates to a misunderstanding of the nature of empowerment. In *The 3 Keys to Empowerment* the authors instruct us to "create autonomy through boundaries" (Blanchard, Carlos, and Randolph, 1999, p. 11). On the surface, this may sound contradictory, but boundaries are not meant to squelch autonomy. Instead, they are parameters—guidelines within which people can safely operate. In explaining this concept, I often remind people that a driver's license gives us the right to travel wherever we would like, but we still have to stop for red lights. Empowerment, therefore, is not chaos, but a framework that gives people the power to make safe and effective choices.

As dementia progresses, people develop increasing difficulty with initiation (starting an activity), sequencing (performing the parts of a task in the correct order), and executive function (planning and problem solving). Therefore, care partners may need to help them get started, cue them through each step of an activity, and help them to figure out why something may not have gone as they planned.

This is the framework the care partner provides. Within this framework, however, a degree of autonomy must be maintained so as not to disempower and discourage the person. For example, if a person is having trouble figuring out which buttons go with which buttonholes, it is helpful to point out the correct match, but it is important to resist the urge to go ahead and do the buttoning.

It takes a fair amount of trial and error to determine how much structure each person needs and what types of choices he can still make for himself. The key is to avoid either the extreme of taking away all independence or leaving him with so many choices that he is overwhelmed. There are no hard-and-fast rules. The correct answers flow from individualized, relationship-based care.

In other community environments, such as assisted living, the same transformational principles apply as those listed for private homes and nursing homes. The assisted living environments that are currently available tend to have several characteristic shortcomings. First, the physical designs are looking less and less like a home and more like a luxury hotel. While they may look very nice, there is nothing in such an environment that provides comfort, familiarity, or meaning for a person with dementia who has left her own home. The interior design may look quite attractive and yet be totally foreign to the type of lay-out, decorations, or furnishings people might have in their own homes.

Second, staffing patterns may be just as haphazard in assisted living as they are in many nursing homes, disrupting the formation of meaningful relationships. Finally, the same balance between providing structure and enabling a degree of autonomy is often missing. I often see people move to assisted living environments that are advertised as "designed for dementia," and they do very poorly. The building is attractive, all of the wander alarms are in place, and there is targeted dementia-specific activity programming, but individual needs are often overlooked. Moreover, between the activity periods, people with dementia are usually "left to their own devices," without the structure and cueing they need to engage in a meaningful way. As a result, there is a tendency for many people in these environments to withdraw and become isolated or else to become anxious or agitated, beginning the cycle of overmedication and decline. The irony is that in a rush to provide alternatives to nursing homes, we often create other environments that are no better at meeting the individual needs of the person who lives with dementia.

Hospitalization

When people with dementia are admitted to the hospital, their situation is especially precarious. Many people leave the hospital in a more confused and less functionally able state than before they became ill. There are several reasons for this.

First, any move to an unfamiliar environment can be disorienting and distressing for a person with dementia. On top of that, there is an acute illness or injury that necessitates the move. Therefore, it is likely that there is also a component of pain, respiratory distress, and/or delirium.

All of the drawbacks of the institutional care environment exist in greater quantity in a hospital setting. There is no time or opportunity to develop close relationships with staff. Autonomy and choice are all but eliminated in the setting of acute care. There are fewer activities or opportunities for one-on-one interaction. Sleep patterns are disrupted by frequent blood pressure checks, treatments, and overall commotion.

Because the dangers of prolonged hospitalization are well known, there is a desire to minimize the length of the hospital stay. While this is an admirable plan, it carries some additional consequences. New medications may be piled on more quickly, or in higher doses. People are more likely to be connected to IV lines and bladder catheters. Any person who impedes the diagnosis and treatment process is likely to be countered with sedation and physical restraints.

Clearly there is no easy way to make hospitalization safe for people with dementia. There are some general principles, however, that can minimize the toxicity of the environment. The first is to use as much stable staffing as possible. As in any care environment, familiar faces can help calm an anxious person, and dedicated staff members have a better understanding of the needs of the individual in distress. Nighttime should be as quiet and uninterrupted as possible. Practitioners should ask themselves whether those blood pressure and temperature checks really need to happen as often as every 2 to 4 hours at night.

Daytime care should allow for sunlight exposure, walking, or other activity, according to the person's level of ability. All of the issues of lighting and environmental noise already discussed apply to the hospital as well. From a medical standpoint, there are several other considerations. Medications should be minimized—don't use three different antibiotics or two different pain pills where one will do the job. It is especially important to avoid those medications with anticholinergic properties, as will be described in Chapter 11.

Another problem lies in the many "lines" that get attached to each hospital patient. Dr. Richard Sterns, chief of medicine at Rochester General Hospital, used to say, "Something strange happens when people get admitted to a hospital: they must forget how to drink and pee, because they all automatically get an IV and a catheter!" Each device acts as an additional irritant for anyone who is confused, distressed, or feeling threatened.

For that reason, we should only attach these devices to people who need them, and we should remove them as soon as the person can manage without them. If the person can take fluids and pills by mouth, the IV can be stopped (or else changed to a heparin lock or a peripherally inserted central catheter, if intermittent doses of medicine are still required).

It is generally better to bathe and use absorbent products with a person who is frequently incontinent than to leave a catheter in for several days. The catheter is a source of pain and irritation and is more likely to cause bleeding and infection over time. Physical restraints should be avoided if at all possible. They generally increase the level of one's distress and therefore the risk of injury. Many people in hospitals and nursing homes have died from strangulation or asphyxiation caused by struggling with restraints.

Delirium without severe emotional distress should be addressed by treating the underlying cause. If severe distress complicates a hospitalization, an antipsychotic pill may be needed for a short time, but the minimum effective dose should be used and the drug tapered off when the condition resolves. In the case of delirium, other types of psychiatric drugs are of no value and should be avoided.

Once the risks have been minimized, the person should be discharged to another care environment as soon as he is stable enough to be treated elsewhere. If he is not well enough to return to the community, a short stay in a nursing home is generally preferable to more days in the hospital.

Finally, staff should use the techniques for communication, interaction, responding to, and investigating distress outlined in Chapters 9 through 13. The basics of interpersonal interaction are too often overlooked in the acute care setting but are no less important.

CHAPTER 7

Bingo and Bird Funerals

Meaning and Activity in Daily Life

CHAPTER 4 DISCUSSED how the institutional approach to care strips meaning from people's daily lives. Time studies of traditional nursing homes have shown that daily life usually consists of medical interventions, meals, and programmed activities, separated by long periods of doing little or nothing. This is especially evident in people with dementia (Perrin, 1997).

This chapter begins by detailing the ways to enrich daily life, because many organizations that pursue culture change fail to fully realize this aspect of transformation. Once again, the prototype is the nursing home, but life at home or in other community settings can be just as devoid of meaning, especially for those who live with dementia.

Creating Meaning

Walk around your own home or apartment. What do you see that holds meaning for you? There are probably a lot of things: photos, special possessions, favorite clothing or jewelry, plants, pets, even family members. Another aspect of meaning is the personalization of your own living space. Then there are the less tangible aspects of meaning: being able to decide when you eat, sleep, and wake, and what you will do throughout the day. Meaning can also be found in the relationships you have with the people who share your space, and the history and stories your home holds for you.

Now walk around a traditional nursing home. Where is the meaning for the people who live there? Is there any in the lounge, the nurses' station, the dining room? Usually what little meaning the elders have is crammed into their bedroom (or half a bedroom).

The less tangible aspects of meaning are also missing, and often more dearly missed: the lack of control and the lack of connection to, or relationship with, those who share your living area. Is it any wonder that people with dementia wander about, or repeatedly say they want to go home?

> The operative logic is the plan that organizes the day in an effective, purposeful, rational, and systemic way: nursing plans; meal plans; seating plans; plans for breaks, communication, rest, sleep—you name it! The systemic element implies that every person is a replaceable entity within the matrix. The individual's point of view is excluded. (Innes, 2003, p. 62)

Community housing developments can create a more subtle loss of meaning. Many such facilities are beautifully landscaped and decorated, but does the design hold meaning for you? Does it reflect your personal style? How much can you personalize the living space? And do you have meaningful relationships with the other people in the community? Does the range of daily activities reflect your own individuality? In our educational workshops, we often ask, "If someone switched the activity calendars from two of your communities, would anyone be able to tell the difference?"

Even in their own home, a diagnosis of dementia can deprive people of the ability to decide how their days are spent. Their activity can be reduced to staring out the window or at a television screen because their care partners may not understand how to maintain and foster engagement through the changes they experience with dementia. As the details of personal history become lost to a person with dementia, *meaning must also be created in the present moment.*

One of the greatest problems with institutional care is the manner in which important rituals are turned into meaningless routines. There is no better example of this than the dining experience. In the institutional model, food is prepared far from the people who live there and transported on plastic trays. Everyone is gathered together and the "trays are passed," food and plastic wear are unwrapped, and drink containers are opened. Then things get even worse.

In the traditional family, mealtime usually takes on a central, almost mythical role. Imagine our own family rituals: perhaps a blessing of the food, a sharing of the events of the day, and discussion of upcoming plans. We even chuckle at the way our parents would admonish us to eat our vegetables before our dessert, or keep us mindful of "starving children around the world" whenever we turned up our noses at the plates before us.

How often is there some sort of ritual greeting or acknowledgment of the act of gathering together at a nursing home meal? Is there meaningful connection and conversation, or do people sit in silence as forkfuls of food are dispensed to those who cannot feed themselves? Is everyone on a schedule? Is there time for those who wish to linger over each bite, or who take a bit longer to chew and swallow?

One of the most important events of the day becomes a kind of drill—a forced march. The person who wants to eat alone in her room may be seen as being antisocial, when in fact she may simply be trying to create some sacred space around this important activity.

In designing the Green House® model (Thomas, 2004), a central goal was a return to the philosophy of *convivium*, an old Roman term for "sharing good food with people we know well" (p. 265). But even in a traditional nursing home, one can create a more convivial and meaningful experience by rethinking mealtime. The key is not just to provide nutrition and calories, but also to create a dining *experience*, rich with engagement and reflective of the individuals who partake in the meal.

The mealtime ritual is more than a simple routine. There is usually a defined beginning, a welcoming of the people gathered around. This might be a blessing of the food, but the welcome need not be rooted in a particular religious ideology. The ritual may proceed in a characteristic way, much like routines do. The difference is the inclusion of all into the process and the presence of active engagement. Whereas routines are built upon sequenced steps, rituals are built on relationships.

Inclusion also means accommodating different styles and pace. Rituals are about the experience, not the schedule. Finally, rituals usually have a closing. It need not be formal, but people do not usually leave the event without their presence being acknowledged and their participation appreciated.

If mealtime is important to people, holiday meals and celebrations are even more so. Adding the traditions and meaning of a holiday gathering to the process of sharing food with people close to you takes on a special sacredness. Indeed, the holidays themselves often get too much of a generic approach in communal living environments, which can ultimately destroy their meaning.

In the film *The Savages* (2007), estranged siblings are forced to confront their father's dementia and move him to a nursing home. There are many images of the nursing home throughout the movie, but one of my favorites is a brief transitional scene used to denote the passage of time. In the shot, we see a bulletin board with a picture of a turkey attached. An employee reaches up, roughly pulls down the turkey, and staples a Santa Claus in its place.

How often do we mark the passage of time with cute holiday decorations, but without exploring the meaning of each holiday for the people who now share this living space? We don't all celebrate each holiday the same way, any more than we dress the same way or listen to the same music.

Last December, our neighborhood teams engaged in an exercise in which we asked all individuals living in the neighborhood to tell us what holiday they celebrated that month, how they celebrated it, and what special memories they had of years past. We asked the same questions of the staff on the team. Then we worked together to create a celebration that would be more unique to the individuals who lived and worked there, and not just a generic occasion.

While we may not have been able to re-create every special moment for every person, what resulted was a better connection with the true essence of the holidays for each person. One Polish gentleman with advanced dementia responded to our questions by saying that he hadn't had an authentic Polish sausage dinner since he moved in. Concerns about his swallowing had limited his food choices. With the blessing of the dietitian, we cooked Polish sausage with apples and sauerkraut in a slow cooker; he ate more than he had in weeks, and his neighbors enjoyed the special meal as well.

Another important event that can become profaned in the institutional environment is death. The pressing need for nursing homes to provide rooms for people who are waiting in hospital rooms or in the community forces a fast-paced admission process that leaves little space for grief or remembrance. Care partners barely have time to pause and reflect before a new person arrives with new needs. Needless to say, this is a process directly at odds with the philosophy of developing close relationships.

Another underappreciated factor is the impact of this process on others who reside in the home. Our institutional approach is usually to "protect" other residents from the death of a neighbor. It is not uncommon to remove the deceased while others are occupied, at mealtime or elsewhere, and to park the hearse by a rear door or loading dock.

Leaders in culture change see these disparities for what they are—an abandonment of the principles of care that guided the person through life, only to be left behind after the last breath is taken. They recognize that unresolved grief tears at the fabric of the community they are seeking to create.

Several years ago, Reverend Julie Berndt saw these disparities in the way death was handled at a Rochester, New York, nursing home. She felt that something more visible and available to all should be offered at the time of death. She also knew that it could be an emotion-laden topic to raise in a nursing home.

In the 2000 Pioneer Network conference, Reverend Berndt recalled approaching the elders at the home with more than a little trepidation. She explained carefully that she was uneasy with the way death was hidden away in normal practice. She felt that something more should be done so that all could pay tribute to the departed. When one of the women in the room began to cry, Reverend Berndt became concerned that she had been insensitive in her comments. The woman, however, reassured her that she was crying from relief. She had been aware of how death was handled at the home, and was afraid that when she died, no one would acknowledge or remember her.

With the blessing of the elders, the home embarked on a new ritual of respect for the deceased. Now when a person dies, a bell is rung three times over the public address system (the only occasion when it is used in the home), and the person's name is quietly announced. Staff and elders alike are welcome to visit the person's room, and bedside prayers are offered. Then all who wish form a procession to the front door, escorting the deceased, who is draped with a meaningful item, such as a favorite blanket or a flag.

When families keep vigil at a nursing home, it is not uncommon for a person with dementia to attempt to enter the room, often appearing distraught. Many such people have lost their ability to communicate their needs verbally. This is commonly interpreted as confused behavior and the person is quickly removed to another location, so as not to upset the grieving family. What often goes unrecognized is that even people with severe dementia may sense the imminent passing of a neighbor, and they may approach the room in their own attempt to process the event. Their feelings of grief are often seen as agitation and swept aside, without allowing them to reconcile the loss.

Care partners need to recognize this for what it represents and help these individuals pay respect to the dying and process their loss. To the extent that a brief bedside visit is feasible, it can greatly allay a person's anxiety. If the family is not receptive to this, a care partner should accompany the person to a quiet place and use validation or a quiet presence to help the person process her emotions in a safe and accepting manner.

After the death of anyone in a nursing home, there is immense value in finding time for members of the community to come together and remember the departed. A few words from staff or other elders can provide closure and can reassure each person that he or she is cared for and will be remembered. This is hard work in the hectic day-to-day pace of long-term care, but it is essential to the creation of a caring community.

A Most Unusual Funeral

People with dementia are keenly aware of loss in their lives. Some of these losses are much greater than their care partners might anticipate, but they need to be recognized as such.

Dierdre lived at St. John's Home and had a pet bird that accompanied her to the home after her husband's death. She had an elaborate daily routine of feeding "Birdie" and cleaning his cage, covering it at night and kissing him through the cage bars. One day, Birdie was found dead on the floor of the cage. Cyndy Hanks, the nurse manager, told me that Dierdre became inconsolable as a result of this loss.

To the credit of her care partners, Dierdre's loss was recognized and acknowledged. She was treated with compassion, and many condolences were given for her loss. With the help of our Spiritual Care department, a memorial service was held in Birdie's honor. The pastor wrote a special remembrance, and the staff created an appropriate vessel, described by Cyndy as "a small wicker basket, lined with a wee soft mattress and quilt topper, and decorated with ribbons." When it was time, all staff and elders were invited to attend the service, which was held right in the neighborhood so that nobody was excluded. The pastor wore a full robe and brought a decorated portable altar. Dierdre's niece also attended. A CD of bird songs and other nature sounds provided a backdrop. The message, as Cyndy related, was "We love you and we share your loss." After that, Dierdre was able to move on.

In the preceding story, the fact that Dierdre and her bird were forced to move to St. John's Home after her husband's death was not lost on her care partners. The symbolic importance of her bird cannot be over-stated. Cheston and Bender (1999) have written about "transitional objects" (p. 226), which may be as varied as a pet, a stuffed animal, a photograph, or an article of clothing. These objects maintain a connection to an "attachment figure" from earlier life and help the person to adjust to a new and unfamiliar environment. The loss of such a transitional object as Dierdre's bird could well have rekindled a grief similar to the original loss of her husband. (Cyndy herself passed away in 2008. Her kindness, compassion, and devotion to the elders in her care were an inspiration for all of us.)

One more comment about spirituality: People with advanced dementia are often regarded as being incapable of engaging in spiritual pursuits or unable to partake in religious ceremonies and observances. Bryden (2005) challenges this assumption:

> In the face of declining cognition, and increasing emotional sensitivity, spirituality can flourish as an important source of identity. And yet the stigma that surrounds dementia may lead to restrictions on our ability to develop our spirituality. It threatens our spiritual identity. . . . Is cognition the only measure of our presence among you as spiritual beings? . . . For you to connect to us spirit to spirit at this level requires sensitivity to what gives us a sense of meaning, what faith tradition, what ritual, what worship practice. Focus on the reality of the present, the simple joy of creation. You can reach across cultures, across faiths, by touching our spirit in ritual, nature, song, music, dance, or other ways to connect us with the ground of all being, the divine. (pp. 150–153)

Subsequent chapters will use the concept of meaning to find new models for behavioral expressions in dementia and to help us understand many of those expressions that our initial investigations fail to elucidate.

Activities

This section turns to the subject of activities for people with dementia. There are enough books on various activity approaches to fill a library, and a book such as this could never do them all justice. A few creative approaches to communication will be discussed in Chapter 10. Rather than try to summarize the vast array of activities, however, I will take a different approach in this book. It would be far more useful here to outline some important principles that should be applied across *all* activities, whether spontaneous or as part of a therapeutic recreation program:

1. *There is much more to life than programmed activities.* There is no doubt that large-scale programmed activities help enrich our lives. Who doesn't enjoy a movie, concert, or sporting event? However, adding more programmed activities does not fill the emptiness in the lives of people in institutional settings. Such activities, though enjoyable, are mainly entertainment. A person's life must also be rich with engagement and individual meaning.

   The secret, then, is not to add more movies or bingo games to the nursing home calendar; they are valuable and enjoyable, but there are plenty of them already. Instead, we need to fill the other spaces of the day with meaningful engagement.

2. *Therefore, each interaction should be as rich with engagement and individual meaning as possible.* This means that each activity should maximize its connection with the unique individuals who are involved. This takes into account their life history, likes and dislikes, work history and hobbies, religion, and values. It also takes into account their cognitive and functional abilities and their particular needs regarding the environment surrounding the activity.

   This also applies to interactions that are not usually thought of as activities, such as mealtime, personal care, and nursing treatments. Keep in mind that such engagement is more than simply informing someone of what you are doing; it is a give-and-take, a sharing of stories. Remember that meaning flows from relationships.

3. *Focus on abilities, not disabilities.* By taking into account a person's existing strengths and by using creativity, people can gain a feeling of inclusion and accomplishment. While a mismatch between an activity level and one's cognitive ability may lead to frustration or anger, it is important not to sell people short without trying to include them. Sometimes there are keys to unlock memories and abilities thought to have been lost.

   In her book *Inside Alzheimer's: How to Hear and Honor Connections with a Person Who Has Dementia* (2007), Nancy Pearce tells the story of Freda, a woman who was viewed as disruptive because she spent most of the day shouting, "Come 'ere, come 'ere, come 'ere" to anyone who was within earshot. She never expressed coherent thoughts and was felt to be incapable of doing so.

Because Freda seemed a bit calmer in the presence of others, Pearce brought her into a group activity, much to the distress of the other people, who felt she did not belong and would disrupt the conversation. Pearce had brought a variety of colored papers and the group was describing the colors and what they meant to them. Freda seemed to watch attentively. After holding up a green sheet of paper and eliciting comments from the group, Pearce turned to Freda expectantly and asked her to share her thoughts.

Freda replied, "Green is the color of a wedding banquet in Bridgeport with flowers and greenery that were so luscious they could have been eaten." Pearce commented on such "islands of clarity," stating, "These precious moments present themselves more frequently when the person with dementia is with someone who is relaxed, open and non-judgmentally present" (pp. 62–63).

Theresa Hart-Piedmont, a music therapist at St. John's Home, also shared two experiences when a perceived mismatch resulted in a positive benefit. In the first story, Donald began attending her music therapy sessions, but his abilities did not match those of the other participants. He was unable to engage as the others did, but he seemed attentive and appeared to enjoy himself. Through one-on-one conversation, Theresa was able to find out from Donald that he used to enjoy playing a phonograph at home, and he often opened his window and shared his music with his neighbors. This was a very important memory for him. Theresa was able to get a phonograph and some old record albums, and Donald now spends many an afternoon acting as "deejay" and playing songs for his neighbors at St. John's.

On another occasion, a woman who had never made any coherent remarks to her care partners was brought to the room. She sat silently in the recliner while the others shared patriotic songs. When Theresa attempted to end the session, one of the participants kept on going, striking up an *a capella* version of the "Battle Hymn of the Republic." As Theresa struggled to find her key and play along, she suddenly heard her "silent participant" joining in on the song. Through one old song, a connection had been made that had not existed before.

4. *Ritualize the activity.* As already discussed, the components of a ritual can be applied to any activity to make it more meaningful for the participants. Therefore, an official welcome will help each participant feel valued and included. This feeling of value also extends to how one is invited to the activity. It is common for care partners to say to a person with dementia, "We're going to have a gathering with some tea and cookies. Would you like to come?" While this is very cordial, it often does not elicit the answer one would like. Being asked to make a choice to attend can be difficult for a person with dementia. What is it all about? Will I know anyone? What will be expected of me? Will I be asked to do or say things that I cannot remember how to do or say? If the person is in a relatively comfortable place, she may be unwilling to risk going to an activity that might be uncomfortable. Conversely, if a person is in distress (even though the activity might be the perfect remedy), her inability to make such a choice may be magnified further.

   Kuhn and Verity (2008) recommend rephrasing the request into an *invitation*:

   > Instead of asking, "Would you like . . . ?" you say, "Earl, I have come to invite you to an outing. I would like you to be my guest." Think about the difference between being asked versus being invited. An invitation implies that you are special and that you are needed. It implies a relationship and an activity that is important to you. An invitation is associated with good feelings so that a positive response is likely. Keep in mind that it is not enough to get the wording right—you need to truly mean what you say when you extend an invitation. (p. 45)

5. *Express gratitude for his or her participation.* The final link in the chain of self-esteem is to appreciate the person. Thank him for his presence and his contributions, no matter how small. Sarah Rowan, in telling her husband's story, instructs care partners that "each activity must celebrate the person with dementia."

6. *Don't forget the value of "being."* Chapter 4 discussed how traditional care environments tend to follow the values of younger adults, whose focus is on "doing." The chapter also reviewed Thomas's characterization of elderhood as a separate, "being-rich" developmental stage.

   Even though aging may slow a person's step or speech, it creates space to appreciate those states of being that are often underappreciated by younger people. We must remember not to be so focused on "keeping people busy" that we forget to tune in to those opportunities for connection that can run so much deeper than what we accomplish with ordinary "doing" activities.

Many people who volunteer to spend time with people with dementia have a lot of anxiety about what to say or do. Sometimes the easiest and best way to start is simply by being with a person. Share a sensory experience: listen to music, watch the children playing on the playground, put your four hands into a soil-filled planter, or drink a cup of coffee and watch the sunset.

This approach also works in many instances when a person is distressed. It helps the person to center himself, block out distractions, and quiet those disturbing thoughts. Often the experience will trigger thoughts and memories that would have been inaccessible had you tried to ask directly. Some of the most magical moments can appear unexpectedly during a time of quiet reflection. Because people with advanced dementia remain incredibly tied into states of being, they can often share this experience in return. My colleague, Diane Hecht, NP, told me this story from her days at another nursing home in Rochester:

> Winnie was a friendly and humorous woman who lived on a locked unit that was deemed "the behavioral unit."
>
> I first met Winnie in 1998 when she came to the nursing home from her family's home. (She was at a moderately severe stage and had trouble verbalizing her needs.) They were unable to care for her at home because of wandering at night and episodes of aggression.
>
> Her family was very loving and shared with our staff that she was a wonderful mother and grandmother. She was cherished for many qualities, especially singing babies to sleep and her incredible baking skills.
>
> When an elder on the unit cried or called out, she at times would also become distressed, but there were times when staff would find her holding the hand of a peer who was distressed and singing softly to them. The calming effect she had was profound.
>
> I recall during one of our many culture change group gatherings of 8 to 10 people, including staff, elders, and family members, she again showed us her kindheartedness. A member of our group, Daniel, was a 54-year-old man who had had a stroke with a "locked-in syndrome." He could only communicate with his eye movements, up or down, and of course with tears.
>
> The group was discussing family, home, and memories,

when Daniel began to cry. His wife was holding his hand, and Winnie maneuvered her wheelchair across our formed circle over to Daniel. She hummed to him softly and held his other hand. Our group, especially Daniel's wife, was touched by her actions.

We as a group recognized that the concept of *peer caregivers* was an untapped resource. The fear of having an elder with "behaviors" interacting with other people from other "units" (as we still called them) was discussed at length. What blossomed from that discussion was a self-selected group of five caring elders who resided at the nursing home and who were committed to learning the basics of dementia and comforting a peer.

This story is a classic example of what our standardized cognitive scales miss when they evaluate people with dementia. Sabat (2001) pointed to research that shows that Alzheimer's disease often spares the prefrontal cortex, an area of the brain that helps people to "behave in socially sensitive ways toward others" (p. 271).

Sabat remarks that "displays of love, affection, friendship, and humor are far more complex than are many of the functions that are examined on neuropsychological tests," and that these traits "should be valued as highly when assessing the cognitive abilities" of those with dementia (p. 269). Further on, Sabat gives a list of abilities that are often preserved into advanced stages of dementia. These include experiencing pride and maintaining dignity, as well as experiencing shame and embarrassment, feeling concern for others, communicating feelings with assistance from a facilitator or by using nonverbal aids, maintaining self-esteem, and manifesting spiritual awareness. Sabat adds, "It is ironic that while many of these capacities are highly valued by the human community, they remain unexamined and unaccounted for in assessments of cognitive function" (p. 322). I have seen people with a Mini-Mental State Exam score of 0 out of 30 who can nevertheless recognize distress in another person and provide comfort to him. What do we do to acknowledge that precious gift?

Enhancing the Experience of Concerts

Before closing this chapter, I would like to reflect on my own experience as a musician and performer. I regularly sing and play for the people at St. John's Home and for others whom I meet in my travels. While entertainment can be fun, there are ways to enhance the experience that all performers should consider in such care settings. Here is my "12-Step Program" for sharing music:

1. *Sing*, and encourage others to join in. Use a lot of sing-along tunes to get people involved. The act of singing is also good for the lungs and for one's overall mood.

2. *Play*, and encourage others to join in—with percussion instruments or hand clapping.

3. *Dance and move*, encouraging physical expression of the rhythms you provide.

4. *Laugh, cry, and feel.* I like to mix moods in my choice of songs. Help people to experience a range of emotions.

5. *Share universal experiences.* Choose songs that speak to common experiences to increase connection to the music. (The song "Five Constipated Men" is a huge hit with the nursing home crowd. Don't ask.)

6. *Play something old.* Even people with longstanding dementia remember old-time melodies. These songs can trigger memories and engage people who might otherwise remain detached.

7. *Play something new.* Challenge people with a few new songs and styles, just enough to broaden their experience beyond the old tried-and-true.

8. *Don't coddle.* Don't be afraid to sing songs about aging, love, and loss. Old people know they are old; they know they are mortal. There is a catharsis in expressing all of our feelings in song.

9. *Don't preach.* Try to avoid songs that moralize or tell people what to think. It's a good way to shut people's minds. Better to tell a story in song, and let people make up their own minds.

10. *Improvise.* As we discussed, spontaneity and variety are the spice of life. Once I was giving a concert at St. John's and a group of preschoolers from our childcare center came in and sat in the front. I threw away my song list and started doing children's songs, like "Old MacDonald Had a Farm." The kids got involved and the elders loved the spectacle and joined in. It was much better than the show I had planned.

11. *Use music to heal.* Music has an incredible power to heal the mind, body, and spirit. It can exercise the heart, lungs, and muscles and

increase circulation. It can release endorphins, create togetherness, and bring about reminiscence. It can open pathways once thought lost to disease. And it is good for the care partners as well.

12. *Reach from, and for, the heart.* (No explanation needed.)

———————

To summarize this chapter, there is more to activity than keeping busy. We understand this, and yet we are often blind to these same needs in people with dementia. Once again, this is not just a discussion for nursing homes. As Sabat's stories of Mrs. D. and Mrs. R. illustrated, meaningful engagement can often be lacking in the home as well.

As you evaluate the various activity programs that abound in all care settings, try to apply the deeper principles I have outlined in this chapter. To quote the eminently quotable Tom Kitwood (1997) once more:

> The hallmark of collaboration is that care is not something that is "done to" a person who is cast in a passive role; it is a process in which their own initiative and abilities are involved. (p. 90)

In Chapter 10, I will discuss in detail one program, the Spark of Life, that meets these principles with impressive results that carry over beyond the activity itself. We will also talk a bit about creativity and the arts as a means to facilitate communication.

CHAPTER 8

Death of the Nursing Home?

Aging in Community

As THE NUMBER OF OLDER PEOPLE continues to rise, there is a growing movement that advocates aging in place—staying in one's own home for as long as possible. As we have seen, however, the home can become maladaptive to the needs of older adults, especially those who live with dementia.

In response to this concern, several efforts are under way to help keep people at home safely. The technology sector has been exploding with new adaptations for aging in place. People with physical and cognitive limitations will soon be courted with a variety of devices for their homes: devices that can monitor pill taking, check each time the refrigerator is opened, remind people what to do when, and even measure vital signs and report them to their physicians and/or family members. While much of this technology holds promise, it can be a double-edged sword. Overdependence on technology can lead to medicalization of the lives of elders, turning the home into a "mini-hospital." It can also encourage further social isolation, which we have seen is detrimental to health, cognition, and overall quality of life.

This chapter will look at some new approaches to aging in community that mitigate some of the hazards of aging in place.

The Aging-in-Place Dilemma

Part of the aging-in-place argument centers on our escalating health care costs. But will the introduction of all of this technology into the home lower overall costs, especially if health outcomes are not improved? Another concern is the potential for invasion of privacy in a heavily monitored home. Furthermore, the medicalization of home life may leave only a pale imitation of what made one's home a home. Culture change advocates often bristle at advertisements that describe nursing homes as "home-like," as the term suggests artificiality. Now, it seems, we are even making one's own home home-like. Is that what we want?

Eden founder Dr. William Thomas sees the aging-in-place movement as being hampered by another limiting paradigm—that of *linear aging* (Thomas, 2008). Linear aging views the aging process as a continuum between two outcomes: dependence and independence. Each of these outcomes is skewed by our societal prejudices regarding aging. Much of our society views dependence in a very negative light. It is seen as a failure on the part of the individual to manage on his own. A central myth of dependence is that it means relying upon others for life's basic necessities. The dependent person, therefore, is a burden. Our solution for dependence is institutional care.

At the other end of the spectrum is independence, which is idealized by society. Independence often determines our self-worth and our worth in the eyes of others. Our definition of success, therefore, is to rely on others as little as possible. The aging-in-place movement is driven by this paradigm.

This linear view, however, creates a no-win situation. There is a push for absolute independence that leads people to stay in suboptimal living situations. There is also a public dread of institutional long-term care, and this dread leads our regulatory system to respond by turning the nursing home into an even more regulated and disempowering living environment.

Aging in Community

A new paradigm challenges the myths of the linear aging view. This paradigm states that, as humans, we are all dependent on others to some extent. Quality of life is not determined by the presence or absence of dependence, but rather by the form this reliance takes. True well-being, then, resides in having the choice to define *how* we rely on others, not to avoid it altogether.

This new paradigm moves us away from the linear aging view by introducing the alternative concept of *inter*dependence. Thomas (2008) defines this term in the following manner:

> As human beings, we live by and through ceaseless cooperation with others—it is our destiny. The nature of our cooperation with and relationship to others changes as we grow, mature, and then age. These relationships form the foundation of all communities.

This new paradigm moves us away from the notion of aging in place toward a new concept: *aging in community*. This not only acknowledges the reality of our interdependence, but it also takes into account emerging evidence of the importance of social capital. Aging in community is a concept that allows us to move away from the linear aging view and find new approaches to successful aging. These solutions have been slowly evolving over the past few decades, and recent advances should encourage even more innovation.

An example of early progress along this path can be seen in the way the nursing home population has changed over the past few decades. When I began to work in nursing homes, it was not uncommon for many people to move there simply because they needed a bit more help and were less mobile. They may have given up their driver's license due to poor vision, or perhaps they needed more help with housekeeping and cooking than they could find at home. However, many community resources have evolved to keep such people out of nursing homes longer. Some of these include the explosion of senior apartments and assisted living complexes; adult day programs that allow family members time to rest and catch up on other obligations; community senior centers that provide meals, activity, and socialization; and the Program of All-Inclusive Care for the Elderly (PACE)— capitated insurance programs that help keep frail people out of hospitals and nursing homes through a combination of house calls, day programs, and enhanced social services.

Another recent development is the Naturally Occurring Retirement Community (NORC). The NORC is driven by the community rather than by a regulatory, insurance, or health care entity. A "neighborhood" (which might be a street, group of streets, or apartment complex) has several older members and therefore forms a cooperative network for them to assist each other to remain in that community.

Neighbors may help each other with transportation, property maintenance, shared meals, or other services. They may establish a system of "checking in" on each other, with a mechanism for helping out in emergencies. Because these are "naturally occurring" communities, they are driven by the individuals' needs and the collective cooperation of the neighborhood and not pigeonholed into a generic insurance program.

It should be mentioned that much of this movement in the United States is driven not only by the desire to avoid nursing homes, but also by the desire to avoid moving to senior apartments and assisted living (for reasons discussed in Chapters 6 and 7).

Long before these concepts began to take hold in the United States, however, the "intentional community" has been an important part of other societies around the world. Thomas (2008) defines an intentional community as "a group of unrelated people who come together voluntarily to share the rhythms of daily life, in pursuit of some noble aim" (such as environmental sustainability, sharing of community resources, or care of frail elders).

Denmark has been a leader in the cohousing movement for decades. The residents of cohousing communities live in private homes or apartments but share some common facilities and work cooperatively to maintain a neighborhood that is close-knit, interdependent, and often environmentally sustainable.

Multigenerational communities weave the lives of elders into every aspect of community and often incorporate nursing home care into that community as well. Strem (in Burgenland, eastern Austria), a village of 900 people, has been planned as a "village for generations." It was created around a nursing home and assisted living facility and offers housing to many of the employees with an infrastructure of schools, stores, banks, and a post office. Many of the community facilities in Strem have shared use, and the elders of the community remain in close connection with the rest of the village. The care home has a chapel and houses the village concert hall; villagers come to the care home for entertainment, and the elders can participate and have a short walk "home." This design has allowed the region to deal with the challenges of an aging population, and an influx of younger people into the village has reversed the youth migration that other small towns have seen.

In Gojikara Village, a continuing care retirement community in Japan, community design facilitates close interaction among all members while respecting individuality and diversity. In addition, there are "planned inefficiencies" incorporated into the village design, such as winding paths that lead to remote parking spaces. This philosophy helps to highlight the imperfection of normal life and prevent the introduction of efficiencies that can lead to institutional thinking.

Some of these concepts have begun to take root in the United States in the form of multigenerational communities. Although a thorough discussion is beyond the scope of this book, there are a few cautions to be mentioned here. Just as many nursing homes use artificial trappings to imitate culture change, many of the communities that advertise the multigenerational concept are poor imitations of true community. Many are gated, allowing only those who are well-off or otherwise discouraging true diversity. Many have separated areas for children and young families—a "you can look, but you can't touch" type of arrangement. Others are simply gimmicks of architectural design that don't truly have the features that foster an enlivened, interactive community. Buyer beware!

Regardless of the form they take, however, the result of all of these changes in community living options has been a change in the people who come to live in nursing homes. The overall average age at St. John's Home (86) has not changed significantly over the past decade, but we now serve a group of people who are more functionally dependent, are more likely to have dementia, or have more complex medical problems than used to be the case. The proportion of people who are in their last year of life is much higher than it used to be, and the number of people who will live with us for 10 to 20 years has greatly diminished. The trend I am describing is not necessarily good or bad. The important factor is whether the living solution individuals attain is best for them, given their unique circumstances.

Friends and coworkers will often ask me for advice about their relatives with dementia. They describe the home situation and ask whether I think the person is ready for a nursing home. Beyond an obvious crisis situation, I usually respond by looking at the person's overall social capital and well-being. Individuals who have been cut off from all social contacts as a result of staying in their home, who are not able to be engaged in meaningful life throughout the day, or whose expressions of need are causing them to be medicated will likely fare better in a good-quality nursing home than they do at home. But what other living option can the aging-in-community movement offer for those who require the level of care and social capital that a nursing home provides that aging in place cannot?

The Green House® Model

Using the principles of the Eden Alternative, Thomas (2004) has created a compelling prototype for aging in community among those with high-level care needs. The Green House follows a process similar to that which was used to deinstitutionalize people with developmental and psychiatric disabilities decades ago.

Green Houses are basically group homes—large, ranch-style houses designed for people who would otherwise live in a nursing home. They are helped by universally trained care partners and a supportive network of clinical and nonclinical staff. Usually 9 or 10 people live in each house, and each person has a private bedroom with private bathroom and shower. There is a large central gathering space with a hearth, an accessible kitchen, and a large table for communal dining. Care is taken to eliminate institutional trappings such as a nurses' station or medication cart. Medications are kept in locked cabinets in each person's room, and the nurses visit the houses for several hours each day to assist with medications, treatments, and care.

The care partners hold the title of *shahbaz* (plural *shahbazim*, which is Persian for *king's falcons*) and are charged to protect, sustain, and nurture the elders in the home. In addition to certification as nursing assistants, shahbazim have training in CPR, first aid, cooking and safe food handling, basic housekeeping and laundry, activities, team decision making, and household management skills. They work with the elders as a collaborative team to drive daily life in the home.

A guide provides administrative oversight and supports the shahbazim and elders through a *servant leadership* approach that enables them to find empowered solutions to day-to-day challenges. In addition to the shahbazim and nurses, there are medical professionals, social workers, dieticians, spiritual care personnel, and various rehabilitation and recreational therapists who visit the house to lend support and skilled care. Most existing Green Houses blend people with and without dementia.

The first four Green Houses opened in 2003 at Traceway Retirement Community in Tupelo, Mississippi. A study of these first houses showed many superior outcomes for residents compared with people who remained in the original building and also with people who lived in a nearby nursing home (Kane, Lum, Cutler, Degenholz, and Yu, 2007). There were significant improvements in several quality-of-life measures, including privacy, autonomy, dignity, relationships, and an overall sense of well-being.

The study also found higher levels of staff and family satisfaction in the Green Houses. Other improvements included less depression and a slower rate of decline in the elders' ability to perform basic activities of daily living. Traceway subsequently built more Green Houses and eliminated the original nursing home.

Subsequent Green Houses in other states have anecdotally reported improved diets, weight gain, fewer behavioral symptoms, and fewer psychotropic medications, though more controlled trials are needed. Many report fewer injuries among staff due to the incorporation of smart technology such as ceiling-mounted lifts. (See the Resources for more information on The Green House Project.)

With funding from the Robert Wood Johnson Foundation, the Green House movement now has projects operating or under development in nearly two dozen states. In response to the success of the Green House model, many other small-house models of care are being developed by other organizations.

St. John's Home is working to be the first organization in the country to move the Green Houses back into neighborhoods around the Greater Rochester area, rather than being on a separate campus. As we move people into 25 or more of these homes around the community, we will transform our existing multistory campus and engage the community with a restaurant, retail shops, educational facilities, and a child care center. The result will truly be aging in community!

The key to success with this model, as noted before, is comprehensive transformation, not only of the physical structure, but of the operational and interpersonal aspects as well. Without sufficient attention to these areas, a small house will be little more than a mini-institution.

Does it seem that this chapter has wandered a bit off topic? Not at all. The key to transforming our care of people with dementia lies in the transformation of aging in society. Our experiential approach will not truly gain traction until we have the social constructs to help support this coming sea change.

––––––––––

The foregoing discussion has several direct applications to the care of people with dementia in all living environments. In the community, maximizing the use of social capital keeps people with dementia and their care partners engaged and connected to society. This engagement occurs on three levels: (1) a micro level, involving close family, friends, and neighbors; (2) an intermediate level, involving churches, clubs, community centers, and other affinity-based organizations; and (3) a macro level, that of the larger community in which they live.

Applying the transformational process to the traditional nursing home can also create an enhanced sense of community, even within the traditional physical structure. The components of relationship, autonomy, meaning, and growth that accompany such transformation create a nurturing interdependence in an environment once devoid of these features. Further evolution to a small-house model, particularly one that is community based, will facilitate further connection with the larger world.

While these are basic human needs that we all share, nowhere are they greater than in people whose ability to satisfy these needs is compromised by an illness such as dementia. Many people have told me over the years that the Eden Alternative and Green House models seem like a good idea for relatively well people, but they feel that people with dementia would benefit far less, if at all. I tell them that, in fact, the opposite is true; the more you have lost in the old model of care, the more you have to regain with the new one.

As we conclude our discussion of aging in community and living environments, I would like to offer a proposal. For many readers, this may be the most challenging section of the entire book.

A Modest Proposal (Regarding Dementia Units)

Dementia Unit, Memory Care Unit, Alzheimer's Unit, Behavioral Unit—a rose by any other name—they are being built and opened at an astonishing rate in nursing homes and community settings alike. Most of the people I have known who work in these areas are incredibly caring, creative, and dedicated people. However, I am going to make an argument for doing away with dementia-specific living environments. I realize that this flies in the face of prevailing opinion worldwide, but I will argue for it nonetheless.

There are many reasons why people build dementia-specific living areas: specialized physical design, specialized staffing, dementia-specific activity programming, lock-down exit systems, isolation of people with behavioral symptoms, and, sadly, the not-infrequent complaints of other elders and their families who don't want "those people" in their living areas. Yet each of these rationales creates significant problems that outweigh any perceived advantages.

Let's begin with the physical design. If the new space doesn't look and feel like a home, it has little or no advantage over the old one. An unfamiliar environment creates unmet needs that are a prominent factor in the genesis of behavioral expressions. As we have seen, the best environments are those that dismantle the institution and re-create home in all of its aspects. It follows that if a specialty area still has long halls, double rooms, nursing stations, alarms, and call bells (not to mention lack of relationship, autonomy, and meaning), it will provide little added benefit.

Who qualifies for your dementia unit? Everyone with dementia? Only people at certain stages of dementia? People with specific behavioral patterns? There are many different models out there. They all pose significant concerns for the people involved. Today, 50% to 80% of the people in most nursing homes have dementia. Having a specialized living area for only some of these people raises the legitimate question of whether their care is of better quality. The presence of a specialty unit often makes others feel like second-class citizens. And in many homes, those with dementia who don't live on the special unit may, in fact, receive inferior care.

Do we want to have staff with expertise in dementia concentrated on these units? The number of people with dementia in all elder care settings is skyrocketing. *Every* nurse, CNA, activity professional, therapist, or social worker needs to understand how to care for people with dementia, whether the person works in assisted living, rehabilitation, home care, or a nursing home.

Another problem with specially programmed units is that each person's condition changes at a different rate. What happens when someone no longer fits the profile for the program? The usual result is "aging out," which means transferring people to another living area when they no longer meet the unit's cognitive or functional criteria. This whole process of moving people to different living areas is incredibly disruptive to elders, families, and staff. Countless hours of staff attention and energy are consumed in dealing with upset families, becoming acquainted with new arrivals, and responding to the increased distress that often results from these moves. A basic rule of caring for people with moderate or severe dementia should be to move them as infrequently as possible. Their new environment may have a similar layout, but the faces are different, the atmosphere is different, care partner bonds are broken, and it will likely be disorienting and upsetting.

What about the person whose dementia reaches a terminal phase, who can no longer communicate her desires and may be actively dying? Will she get moved to a new place in her greatest hour of need? It happens all too frequently in the world of elder care. Such moves also cause severe distress among care partners who have formed strong attachments. Institutional practices such as moving people when their condition changes cause people who work there to suffer as well as those who live there.

But physical and operational concerns aside, there is a larger philosophical concern that, in my mind, trumps all others. What it boils down to is a matter of civil rights. The basic idea of the dementia-specific living area stems from an institutional mindset that places people into an environment largely defined by their disease, not by who they are. It presumes that people with dementia are enough alike that they should share a common living space, and there is an approach to care planning and activities that reflects their illness more than their individuality. Segregating people due to a physical attribute—sound familiar?

Furthermore, there is a deep prejudice in elder care environments that is shared by other elders and families. "People with dementia should have good care—separate, but equal, and not in our neighborhood." This reflects underlying fears and misconceptions about the disease and sells short the potential for growth and engagement that still exists in people with dementia, as surely as it does in someone who is blind or has lost a limb.

I have often seen family members decline having their loved one move to a dementia-specific living area because they don't want her to be "dragged down by being surrounded by others who have dementia." I used to think this was not a valid concern. However, I have come to see several advantages to a more diverse community. People who are more cognitively able can assist with various neighborhood tasks, facilitate discussions, and model many positive interactions for those with dementia. Being of assistance creates caring opportunities for the more able elders. Also, as we have seen, positive social interactions can bring forth the abilities of people with dementia.

Sabat (2001) wrote of the need for people with dementia to be with healthy others in order to create positive "social personae" to connect them to their past attributes. This is an important step in maintaining self-worth throughout cognitive changes. People with unmet needs may certainly express themselves in ways that can be disturbing to others nearby. However, it bothers me to hear someone say that people with certain behavioral expressions should be moved to a dementia unit because "the people there won't notice as much." Disturbing behaviors disturb *everyone*, and it is a classic case of positioning to presume otherwise. Who would more likely be distressed if a person with dementia strolled into their bedroom at 2 a.m.: a person without dementia who can recognize the "visitor" as being confused, or a person dealing with his own confusion, disorientation, and misperceptions of the environment? Which person would feel more threatened? Aside from this, the disruption of the move will likely make any behavioral expressions worse, not better.

Many of the concerns raised about living with people who have dementia reflect one's own fears and misinformation about the condition. The antidotes to these fears are education, a humane approach to behavioral expressions, transformation of the care environment, and the creation of a nurturing, interdependent community.

Even if you don't accept my arguments about dementia units, at the very least we should get rid of the name in all of its forms. Regardless of how enlightened it may look and sound, naming any living area after a disease reveals an institutional mindset that reduces people to their deficits. It also perpetuates the notion that all people with the disease are alike, should be treated alike, and have no personal identity in our eyes.

Let's stop doing "memory care," "Alzheimer's care," or even "dementia care." Let's care for *people* who happen to have dementia.

Dementia and the "Third World": A Global Perspective

According to the Alzheimer's Association (2009), over 60% of people with dementia live in developing countries. This proportion is expected to rise to 71% by 2040. I have attended many talks where the "problem" of increasing populations with dementia in these countries is a cause of much concern. This mirrors much of society's panic regarding the overall aging of the world's population. Much of this talk centers on the "burdens" that these trends will place on our financial and human resources. I recently looked at a fellowship application that asked me to share how my ideas could be put to use to help people in developing countries.

I do not doubt that our evolving demographics will challenge us all in the years ahead; but all of this focus on how "enlightened" societies can help developing countries makes me think of Binta.

> The wonderful, whimsical Oscar-nominated short film *Binta y la Gran Idea* (*Binta and the Grand Idea*, 2004) concerns a child in a small Senegalese village. The villagers have little technology and Binta attends a thatched, one-room school. Life is simple and close to nature. Community is everything.
>
> One day, Binta learns about life in the "other world." She tells her father about the land where people have so many fish that they don't help each other get food, and so much wealth that they guard it with guns. Her father gets a "grand idea" and enlists Binta to help carry it out. They work their way up through local, regional, and national bureaucracies and finally get permission to carry out their grand idea: to adopt a child from America, which they see as an impoverished nation!

So thanks to Binta and her father, here is my "grand idea." The care of people with dementia in our industrialized nations is impoverished in many ways. Maybe we should ask developing nations what *they* can teach *us* about global aging and the care of people with dementia. I'll bet they would have a lot to say.

———————

Now that we have looked at the drawbacks of our biomedical model of dementia and the features of an experiential approach, it is time to put these ideas to practical use. The next several chapters will apply this new model to the care of people with dementia.

We will start by looking at our basic interpersonal interactions and the important effects they can have on the well-being of people with dementia. We will then show how this approach can be applied to episodes of distress and other common behavioral expressions without resorting to potentially harmful medications.

PART 3

Solutions

CHAPTER 9

Face to Face

Basic Interpersonal Approaches

BEFORE ADDRESSING SPECIFIC behavioral expressions, this chapter begins with some general advice for interacting with people who have dementia. Many of the interactions outlined are intuitive in our lives with family and friends but tend to get lost when we don the institutional hat and become *caregivers*. Some of this advice flies in the face of medical and nursing training, which admonishes us to "keep a professional distance" at all times. It also challenges the use of a paternalistic style in dealing with those who live with dementia. Much of the following advice consists of little more than always remembering to honor the basic humanity of the people in your care.

In their groundbreaking book series, beginning with *The Best Friends Approach to Alzheimer's Care* (1997), Bell and Troxel advocate approaching the person with dementia as one would a close friend. This helps move the emphasis from giving care to a "victim" of Alzheimer's to the reciprocal and empowering interactions that define good friendships.

Bell and Troxel list the following "Elements of Friendship" (1997, pp. 46–47):

Friends know each other's history and personality.

Friends do things together.

Friends communicate.

Friends build self-esteem.

Friends laugh often.

Friends are equals.

Friends work at the relationship.

As you will see, the philosophy of this approach resonates with the philosophy and approaches described in the next several chapters. Friendship, after all, requires getting to know a person well, treating him as an individual, valuing him, and appreciating his perspective on life.

The following list of suggestions for basic communication is not meant to be exhaustive. Rather, it should stimulate the reader to look for alternative approaches unique to his or her own care environment that will enhance the lives of those who live and work there.

Communication 101

Knock. Let's start at the door to a person's room. This is where many interactions begin. In the nursing home, the staff's institutional mindset causes them to regard the home as a workplace, their "domain," and it is not uncommon for staff to walk right into the room. Resist that urge. You are entering someone else's bedroom—this is *their* home, not ours. Do people walk right into your home unannounced? Not normally. Start with a knock on the door, then clearly announce yourself, explain your purpose, ask permission to enter, and don't forget to wait for the answer.

Many staff members assume that because they interact with the elder on a daily basis, they will be easily recognized. This is not always the case, due to a combination of cognitive factors and possible problems with lighting, hearing, and vision. It is best, especially in approaching people with moderate dementia or vision loss, to state clearly who you are each time you enter.

Sit. When I visit people in their room, I always try to sit down. There are several reasons for this. First, there is a subtle hierarchical dynamic when a staff member stands over a person. This suggests that power and control rest with the stander, which may intimidate or threaten the person, even if your demeanor is kind. Second, placing yourself at eye level facilitates communication. (In their Spark of Life workshops, Verity and Lee even recommend trying to be slightly *below* eye level, to give the person with dementia a more important position.) The third reason to sit is that it sends the unspoken message that you have time for people to express their needs, and you aren't simply rushing from one room to the next. People who sit are generally perceived as giving more time and attention than those who remain standing.

I have had some very hectic days in nursing homes, but I try to use an approach to my personal visits that I call "the eye of the hurricane." I may rush from floor to floor, scan the charts quickly, and multitask my way through my day, but when I enter an elder's room, I try to create a moment of calm and relaxation where everything else disappears, if only for those few minutes. This demeanor says, "Right now, I am at your disposal. Feel free to share anything you like, and I will try to meet your needs."

Pearce (2007) reminds us that "a person with dementia tends to have very strong antennae; she can feel when we are distracted, or are not fully present for a connection" (p. 18). Pearce adds that "each person has taught me . . . the importance of relaxing into being in the present moment" (p. 39).

Listen. My next bit of advice is "shut up and listen." We usually have an agenda when we enter an elder's space, and their agenda may get swallowed up in our own thoughts unless we create the space for them to express themselves. A common mistake I see with doctors-in-training is the tendency to be so focused on a certain line of questioning that important comments are ignored.

Adjust your pace. It is very important to slow the pace of speech. I have often heard people complain of "staff rushing me all the time." Younger people tend to speak more quickly, and their words may run together. Older people often process information and respond more slowly than younger people. By not allowing the time for such processing, we unintentionally disempower people.

Bryden (2005) recalls that the onset of her dementia created a feeling "as if the world was too fast for me." She adds this advice:

> I operate in a different way to you, and need a different type of interaction, which is slower and more meaningful. . . . I need a restful, calm environment, with no visual or aural distraction, to listen to what you say and to be able to speak to you. (p. 139)

This reflects Kitwood's concept of outpacing (Chapter 4), which can disempower the person with dementia. Sabat (2001) suggests pacing your speech to mimic that of the person you are addressing.

Connect. Most hard-of-hearing people will tell you they do not need for you to speak loudly, just slowly and clearly. The biggest problems occur with consonants at the beginnings and ends of words. Vowels are fairly easy to hear, but the high-pitched consonants are the first sounds that get dropped by the aging ear.

Try this exercise: read a passage from a book aloud, but keep your tongue anchored in the floor of your mouth and don't let your lips or teeth come together as you say the *p*'s, *t*'s, and other consonants. This will give you an idea of how your words can sound to someone with age-related hearing loss.

Eye contact is important, as are nonverbal cues of understanding and encouragement. In fact, as dementia becomes advanced and verbal comprehension becomes diminished, the nonverbal signals we send take precedence. An elder may not understand your words, but your tone of voice and body language speak volumes.

Bryden (2005) offers this advice to those who approach her:

> As we become more emotional and less cognitive, it's the way you talk to us, not what you say, that we will remember. We know the feeling, but we don't know the plot. Your smile, your laugh and your touch are what we will connect with. (p. 138)

Needless to say, the same is also true of an unfriendly, harried, or judgmental demeanor. Taylor (2007) agrees emphatically:

> In fact, if one is to believe all this preaching about treating us with dignity and in ways that enhance our self-esteem, then caregivers' patterns of communication have a profound impact on those for whom they care.
>
> One of the easiest ways for me to become angry is to perceive that someone is treating me like a child. (p. 189)

This last comment was recently confirmed in a study that showed that using infantilizing language with people in nursing homes who have dementia caused significant increases in their resistiveness to personal care (Williams, Herman, Gajewski, and Wilson, 2009). (My only problem with this study is their use of the term *elderspeak*, which demeans the title of *elder*; it is actually baby talk!)

Another technique that can be used to enhance understanding is to combine hand gestures with your words. Sometimes the visual representation, or the combination of words and gestures, is easier for the person to comprehend than your words alone.

Personal Care

When you think about it, it is remarkable that we expect elders in nursing homes to allow strangers to remove their clothing and bathe them, and even more so that they agree. Dementia care pioneer Joanne Rader has spent a great deal of her career teaching the art of sensitive, humane personal care.

One of the first things Rader did in researching personal care was to ask her coworkers to bathe her. This was not a half-hearted role-play of the activity—they removed all of her clothes, put her in a gown, took her to the shower room, and bathed her. Even though she volunteered and knew her staff to be kind, caring people, she felt embarrassed throughout the experience. How many of us would have the courage to try this?

No matter who is the recipient of hands-on care, it must be gentle, well paced, and dignified. The institutional approach is to perform the function as a simple task, as if the elder were an object rather than a person. The water may not be the right temperature, the person may feel overexposed, or the handling may be too rough for dry, sensitive skin. There may be little or no conversation, which can heighten feelings of embarrassment.

For the person with dementia, there may be little or no understanding of what is being done unless it is well explained. The shower may be noisy and the stream of water unsettling. (Rader recently commented to me that the usually pleasant sensation of water running across her face became a distressing one when she was being bathed by another person and couldn't control the process.) Many people with dementia become quite disturbed by the feeling of a stream of water running over them. People are also quite particular about the exact temperature of the water; if it is only a few degrees above or below the preferred temperature it can be quite bothersome. Institutional tubs may also frighten people. After bathing, the towels may be rough, a comb may hurt a tender scalp, and inadequate drying can lead to skin maceration and breakdown.

For any shower or bath, be sure that the air temperature and ambience are optimized. The elder should remain well covered as much as possible during the process. No additional people should be present—ideally, bathing should be a one-to-one experience. There is nothing more discouraging than hearing that "Mr. Jones was so agitated that it took four people to bathe him." If Mr. Jones didn't want one person to bathe him, sending in reinforcements to force the issue is never going to improve his experience and will likely lead to a very bad day for everyone. Better to skip a bath than to leave an indelible memory that could compromise all future care.

Soft lighting and music may help create a more enjoyable experience. Many homes are renovating their tub and shower rooms to create a softer, more relaxing environment. Noninstitutional linens and electric towel warmers are also a great improvement. A moisturizing lotion provides a nice sensation and aroma and is helpful for dry and cracked skin.

The bather should move in a stepwise fashion and explain each step, waiting for comprehension *and acceptance* before proceeding. Many care partners may worry that if they ask permission, the person might refuse. However, we are much more likely to succeed if we ask first, and if we are rebuffed, we would do well to find out why before trying to proceed.

In many cases, people with severe dementia cannot feel safe and calm during a shower or tub bath. In such cases, a bed bath technique has been developed. This allows the person to remain in bed, swaddled in warm blankets, and gently bathed with special no-rinse soap. Warm, wet towels remove the excess soap and dry towels follow for warmth as the person is dressed. The book and video *Bathing without a Battle* is an essential reference for this topic (Barrick, Rader, Hoeffer, Sloane, and Biddle, 2001).

Many people with dementia have little tolerance for long sessions of personal care tasks. In the institutional model, the focus is on completing the tasks as quickly and efficiently as possible so there is little opportunity to rest. Nevertheless, it can save a lot of trouble if care partners break up the routines of such people into small, manageable segments.

The person could arise, put on a housecoat, and have her hair brushed and face washed. After breakfast, there could be oral care and dressing. Bathing may be saved for another part of the day. Each segment will be accompanied by active and affectionate engagement with the person, thus bringing more meaningful interaction into an otherwise mundane routine. Many professional staff will no doubt read these words and say, "That's all very nice, but I don't have time to engage a person that way, with all of the tasks I'm expected to complete in a short period of time." That is the very reason why so much of this book has centered on deep organizational transformation!

Mealtime and other rituals have been explored in Chapter 7. As mentioned, the key is to include engagement, individuality, autonomy, and personal meaning in such events.

Autonomy and Choice

As was discussed earlier, one of the greatest failures of the institutional model is the loss of choice in most aspects of daily life. This is further compounded in people with dementia, as their care partners and family members often position them as being less capable than they actually are. A battery of cognitive tests helps to determine the severity of a person's cognitive deficits. Most of these, like the widely used Folstein Mini-Mental State Exam, consist of a series of questions designed to test specific cognitive realms (attention, orientation, retention, calculation, spatial recognition, etc.). While these tests help delineate the stage and natural history of the illness, they are rather crude indicators of overall functional capacity, as most thinking processes are much more integrative than this. They may also leave people feeling frustrated and ashamed at their inability to answer the questions.

Knowledge versus Wisdom

We often assume that if a person cannot tell us the date or name her children, then more complex cognitive abilities are probably absent. Fortunately, this is not necessarily the case. A study by Florida State University psychologists illustrates this point (Dijkstra, Bourgeois, Youmans, and Hancock, 2006). The researchers interviewed 18 people from a Florida day center who had dementia that was advanced, by traditional measurements. They found that the elders attended poorly and were often incorrect when asked for factual information about their marriage, family members, or church functions. However, when asked for *advice* on the same topics (e.g., "I'm thinking about having children. What kind of advice can you give me on that?"), the same people were much more focused and coherent, and they were eager to share their wisdom on the subject at hand. The researchers also found that the elders' ability to teach a recipe to the researchers was similar to that of elders without dementia. They concluded that the social role of dispensing wisdom and advice helps fulfill a need that allows elders with dementia to tap into fairly complex cognitive processes. Providing these opportunities on an ongoing basis was recommended to "help to break the cycle of learned helplessness and perceived incompetence to communicate and . . . contribute to feelings of self-esteem and well-being" (p. 365).

In order to provide the optimum environment for engagement and growth, we must therefore be very careful not to underestimate people's abilities to choose and to direct their care. This requires constant attention to the many paternalistic interactions that our prior training has taught us to employ with people who have dementia. If many small episodes of disempowerment can lead to withdrawal and disengagement from life, then it stands to reason that we should give people as many opportunities for choice as they are capable of exercising.

There is no choice too small or unimportant to be exercised in creating a positive environment. Our choice of words should always reflect this. For example, instead of saying, "It's time to go to lunch," one could say, "Hello, Mrs. B. It's lunchtime. Would you like me to walk with you to the dining room?" Using simple choices in the act of providing personal care can also defuse some of the agitation experienced by a person with a low tolerance for such activities (e.g., "Would you like to feel fresh and clean? Would you like me to wash your face or your hands first? Is the water warm enough for you?").

Indeed, many of the agitated and aggressive behavioral expressions we see can be traced to lack of control over one's surroundings. Sometimes, when verbal expression is impaired, it requires a great deal of patience and perseverance to enable choice.

Charades

Paul, a former lawyer, had an atypical dementia that may have been a Lewy body form or may have been related to alcohol overuse. He had significant aphasia; he would often start a sentence and then be unable to find the words to finish his thought. His voice was usually loud, regardless of his mood. He spent much of the day in his room, watching old war movies at high volume on his television set.

Because he was a very large man, the staff needed a directive from physical therapy regarding Paul's ability to stand and transfer from bed to chair. However, the day he was seen by the therapist, he flatly refused to attempt any standing. After a few consecutive days of such refusals, he was relegated to a mechanical lift as the "safest" option. Using the lift terrified Paul. He would become visibly agitated and often flailed his arms wildly while being transferred, occasionally striking the staff members.

A former Marine, Paul was usually calmest with male figures, and James was assigned as his primary aide. He was less accommodating with women, especially if they tried to tell him what he should do. His excitement heightened his aphasia, causing poor communication to deteriorate further.

We suspected that Paul was strong enough to stand and pivot without the lift, but he was never willing to try this when the female therapists came around. We therefore planned another evaluation with our senior therapist, Carol, on a day when James and I would both be on hand to help explain the process and smooth things over.

On the appointed day, I explained to Paul about our plans as he was finishing breakfast in his room. He seemed to understand that we wanted him to stand; he seemed agreeable, but he gestured that he planned to finish his breakfast first. So Carol, James, and I waited for what seemed an eternity, as he very slowly and methodically finished each bite of his breakfast. Any attempt to hurry things along was met with resistance. He displayed an almost compulsive attention to this task. James was called away, leaving Carol and me to fend for ourselves.

When he had finally finished every last bit of food and drink, I removed the tray, but he still would not try to stand for us. He began yelling, "No! No!" very persistently and pointing toward the television on his dresser. What followed was a game of charades, with each of us picking up objects on the dresser, opening drawers, holding up socks and other garments, and pushing knobs on the TV in an attempt to decipher his objection. All Paul could do with each attempt was say "No!" and point once again. Occasionally he would pause and shake his head in frustration.

After about 10 minutes of back and forth, we finally deduced that the remote control was sitting in the wrong spot—he wanted it in a very particular position on the top shelf. Once we corrected that, he relaxed and stopped yelling. I asked once again if we could now try having him stand. Immediately, without waiting for our help, Paul stood up from the chair and pivoted onto the edge of the bed all by himself. After that, the use of stand-pivot transfers, at a time when he was relaxed and ready, eliminated the agitation and striking out that were seen with the lift.

This is an example of the lengths one must occasionally go to in order to address unmet needs. In deciphering Paul's predicament, however, we gained a lot of knowledge about his personality and thinking processes. Knowing about Paul's military history helped us to understand his almost obsessive attention to order and detail and gave us valuable clues about his way of viewing the world. Relationship building and careful attention to each person's individuality can often solve a problem that otherwise might be treated with sedating medication.

Individuals with dementia should have the opportunity to prove that they are unable to make a choice rather than care partners simply assuming this to be the case. Even a person with advanced disease should be given a chance to make simple choices, such as which of two shirts to wear, instead of the care partner automatically picking one out. When I take the time to ask, I am often surprised by the result.

Such choices might seem to be too trivial; however, it is often not the actual choice, but *the act of choosing* that makes the difference. And sometimes it is merely the knowledge that you haven't abdicated all control in your life just because you are ill or living in a nursing home.

The Gift

During medical rounds at St. John's, I once visited a woman who had only been with us for a month. She had Alzheimer's disease and found some information difficult to process, but through careful questioning I was able to ascertain that she was feeling well and had no particular concerns.

After examining her, I asked if she was adjusting to her new living situation, and she said that everything was fine. I usually don't stop there, because many people lower their expectations when they enter a nursing home—if it isn't absolutely horrible, they are often grateful. So I asked, "Is there anything you need that you aren't getting?" Once again, she quickly replied, "No, no, everything is fine."

I decided to try one last question: "If you could do anything you wanted to today," what would you like to do?" There was a brief pause, and I realized she might not be capable of answering such an open-ended question. But a much deeper understanding reached her, and her response was as instructive as it was surprising. She broke into a radiant smile, took my hand, and said, "Thank you! Thank you so much! You are so kind!" Then she dismissed me with a look of pure serenity.

It took me a moment to realize what had just happened. I had hoped to try to grant a wish, and had unknowingly given her a much bigger gift. Her joy came, you see, not from choosing a special request, but from hearing that she *could* choose.

Positive Person Work

We have discussed some very basic principles of interaction, including communication, body language, techniques for providing hands-on care, and enlisting the person in exercising choice. Beyond these basic principles, however, there are specific interactions that will further advance the positive experience of people with dementia and foster their growth and engagement.

There are several frameworks for these interactions, from the Spark of Life program to Montessori-based activities for dementia. For the purpose of this discussion, however, let's review the process that Kitwood called "positive person work" (1997).

In addition to identifying 17 forms of *malignant social psychology* (listed in Chapter 4) that undermine personhood in elders with dementia, Kitwood also identified antidotes to these plagues of institutional interaction. These forms of *positive person work* serve to reconnect the elder with dementia to his basic humanity.

Kitwood also believed that an environment filled with these positive interactions could affect the growth of brain cells, and possibly facilitate new connections and adaptations (a process he termed *rementing*). This theory was met with a good deal of skepticism from the medical community, but recent research (including that which shows new neuronal connections in stroke survivors) should force a reexamination of these ideas.

Brooker (2007, pp. 90–95) adapted these ideas to form the following 17 "personal enhancers":

Warmth—demonstrating genuine care, affection, and concern

Holding—providing safety, security, and comfort

Relaxed pace—creating a relaxed atmosphere

Respect—treating the participant as a valued member of society and recognizing the person's experience and age

Acceptance—entering into a relationship based on an attitude of positive regard

Celebration—recognizing, supporting, and taking delight in the skills and achievements of the participant

Acknowledgment—recognizing, accepting, and supporting the person as unique and valuing the person as an individual

Genuineness—being honest and open in a way that is sensitive to needs and feelings

Validation—recognizing and supporting the reality of the person; sensitivity to feeling and emotion take priority

Empowerment—letting go of control and assisting the person to discover or employ abilities and skills

Facilitation—assessing the level of support required and providing it

Enabling—recognizing and encouraging a participant's level of engagement within a frame of reference

Collaboration—treating the person as a full and equal partner in what is happening; consulting and working with the person

Recognition—acknowledging the person's uniqueness; bringing an open and unprejudiced attitude

Including—enabling and encouraging the participant to be and feel included, physically and psychologically

Belonging—providing a sense of acceptance in a particular setting, regardless of abilities and disabilities

Fun—accessing a free, creative way of being, and using and responding to the use of humor

Kitwood (1997) stressed that care partners must be emotionally present and form meaningful connections in order for positive person work to produce results. This echoes Pearce's (2007) advice about being "in the moment" (p. 109).

As care partners become more fluent in the techniques of personal enhancement, they can begin to combine different techniques as each situation dictates. For example, in the preceding story about Paul, we used techniques of recognition, genuineness, and respect in the way we addressed him, explained our purpose, and waited for him to finish breakfast before proceeding. We used collaboration and facilitation to solve the problem of the misplaced remote control. We validated his frustration and apologized for being slow to understand what he was trying to tell us. And when Paul successfully stood, we praised him and celebrated his accomplishment.

Kuhn and Verity (2008, pp. 86–99) describe the contrast between positive and negative interaction as a series of "putdowns and uplifts":

To intimidate versus to empathize

To withhold versus to be compassionate

To accuse versus to understand

To invalidate versus to validate

To infantilize versus to honor

To objectify versus to personalize

To mock versus to pay respect

To stigmatize versus to affirm

To ignore versus to acknowledge

To disempower versus to empower

To disparage versus to boost self-esteem

To deceive versus to support

To impose versus to promote autonomy

To label versus to describe

To disrupt versus to stand back

To banish versus to include

To outpace versus to pace

Though each of these models has its own format and perspective, it should be clear that there is a common philosophy that unites them all. Like Kitwood, Brooker, Verity, and Kuhn, I believe that every small interaction helps create the landscape of experience of a person with dementia. A person may not recall every interaction or the names of the people she encountered, but she will be left with a positive or negative experience, depending on the sum of those interactions.

These very small encounters play a very big role in a person's sense of well-being. The importance of all of these interactions becomes more critical as cognitive function declines and unmet needs emerge.

Verity uses a powerful skit in her presentations, in which she dons a shawl and holds a large paper heart across her chest. On the heart is written "I am lovable." Assuming the role of "Elsa," a woman with dementia, she tells the story of her day in the nursing home. Each scene begins with a moment of pleasure and peace, until a staff member enters the room and makes a disparaging comment, disempowers her, or ignores her needs. After each episode, Verity rips off a piece of the heart until there is nothing left.

CHAPTER 10

Getting Past the Words

Language and Communication

IN THE PREVIOUS CHAPTER, we reviewed some basic interpersonal approaches. However, there is much more to consider when communicating with a person with dementia, including issues with word processing and comprehension, the meanings of words, and nonverbal communication approaches.

As we age, there is a slowing of speech processing in the brain. Even when we fully comprehend what is being said, it may take a bit longer for us to receive the words, process what we hear, and formulate our response. Certain disease states, such as Parkinson's disease, can slow this process even further. The processes of dementia can also produce deficits along this pathway. A person may have trouble understanding what was said (a *receptive* problem) or making a response (an *expressive* problem). Language abilities may vary from day to day and can be affected by the person's emotional state as well.

Sensory defects can also affect one's ability to converse effectively. It is worth repeating here that it is important to be sure that each person is comfortable and able to see and hear you as much as possible if you want to maximize your communication.

Psychologist Albert Mehrabian (1981) is well known for his

analyses of how we communicate. His research shows that, in conversations where emotions and attitudes play an important role, only about 7% of the meaning we glean is communicated through the words themselves. Another 38% is *paralinguistic,* meaning that it is a function of *how* the words are spoken—the tone and inflection of the voice. The remaining 55% comes from facial expression and body language.

As dementia begins to affect one's ability to process spoken words, the nonverbal components become even more important. It is critical that care partners understand this in order to use their full expressive range to communicate effectively. It is also critical to realize that the tone of your voice and facial expressions may be saying more about your message than your actual words. This means that care partners need their own technique for centering and collecting themselves, particularly in distressing situations. In order to promote compassion and concern, your words must be accompanied by a calm tone of voice and a relaxed face and body posture. This is almost impossible to fake when speaking to individuals whose language reception is impaired, as they usually have heightened awareness of nonverbal signals. It is amazing how well a person with severe dementia can detect insincerity or underlying tension in another person.

As such, the transformational pathway demands that we look closely at the subtle dynamics of the care environment. I have worked in nursing homes where a particular living area has experienced a period of staff conflict. This does not have to consist of overt arguments in public areas. Nevertheless, when such conflict exists, the people with dementia who live in these areas predictably display more distress than those who live among more harmonious staff.

There are two keys to helping care partners achieve a positive approach in their daily interactions. The first is to create a strong support system for all who work within a given environment. Although a more detailed discussion is beyond the scope of this book, a system of support for care partners is critical, due to the difficulty of the work they do on a daily basis. The Eden Alternative pathway contains specific tools to create supportive care partnering teams, facilitate communication, and resolve conflict in a manner that validates and respects the people involved.

The second key is for each person to develop a process that helps him or her to achieve a balanced, centered state of mind when things get hectic. There are several approaches, from meditation to deep breathing to biofeedback. The essential element is mindfulness—the ability to exist in the moment and attend to the feelings at hand in a nonjudgmental manner.

The use of words and body language is explored in more depth in the following chapters that deal with specific scenarios. This chapter will focus instead on how to better understand what the person with dementia is trying to communicate *to us*. The chapter concludes with a look at other techniques to enhance interpersonal connection, including the use of creativity and the arts.

Breaking Through Communication Barriers

There are many ways in which language can be affected in dementia. In keeping with a more holistic approach, I will avoid delving into the complex brain anatomy associated with specific language problems. Instead, I will examine these in a more practical way, based on what words we are hearing when we attempt to converse.

The following is my own classification of seven common types of language problems I have encountered: naming and word-finding problems, word substitutions (receptive and expressive), third-person speech, "confabulation," emotional amplification of speech problems, reversion to a prior language, and tangential or "nonsensical" speech. (I put the last in quotes because there may be a sense to the speech—it just may not be obvious right away.)

Let's examine each of these in detail and explore techniques for "getting past the words" and gaining insight into the underlying meaning. It is surprising how much one can understand when some of these speech patterns are decoded.

Naming and Word-Finding Problems

Many people with advancing dementia begin to have trouble finding the name of an object, or the right words to express an idea. This will often appear as nonfluent speech, with hesitations, stammering, and a visible degree of frustration.

Sometimes the person will draw a blank and stop. The person may also gloss over the lost words (e.g., "I was carrying the . . . the . . . um . . . the *thing*, and I dropped it"). In many cases, the person may remember what happened but is unable to find the right word. Doctors may refer to this as dysnomia, anomia, or anomic aphasia—the inability to name things.

It is usually helpful to give the person a bit of space to try to find the words on her own; jumping in too quickly may miss the mark and increase her frustration at being interrupted. However, if the person is clearly struggling and in need of help, it can be useful to help her along with educated guesses.

In some cases, the missing words can be easily guessed by the context of the situation. In the sentence just quoted, if the person is standing over a shattered coffee cup, it is easy to guess what the "thing" was that she dropped. Being centered in our approach helps us to be sensitive to more subtle environmental and emotional cues as well.

Word Substitutions

At times, rather than stumbling over a word, a person might substitute a different word or phrase. There are several forms this may take. Sometimes the word will be related to the intended word: "I was reading the, um, the 'daily'" (meaning "newspaper"). Or it may be a descriptive phrase: "I need, um, the thing you use to pick up the food." The second phrase is fairly obvious to figure out, but the word *daily* might confuse someone who isn't used to hearing such a term. You might repeat the word back for clarification, and see if she can supply another word or description to help you out.

Sometimes the substituted word is incorrect but is related to the intended word: "I have to call my mother" (intending to say "daughter"). We have all done this from time to time. It is important to recognize that this may be a simple substitution, and not jump to the conclusion that a person is confused or even delusional.

Another type of substitution is a word that sounds like the intended word, even a rhyming word: instead of saying, "I lost my purse," she might say, "I lost my perk" or "I lost my curse," which could lead the listener astray. There may also be additional meaning to be gleaned from the chosen word. "The staff threw me to bed," instead of "put me to bed," may suggest an underlying feeling that she was handled roughly in the process.

In each case, you can help clarify the comment by asking her to repeat what she said, by guessing the correct word and asking for confirmation, or by asking for more information. The last approach would be useful in the case of "I lost my perk." You can ask for clarification, or simply say, "Oh, dear. Where was it when you lost it?" Her response might make the lost object clearer to you: "I took it out to get money for the ice cream shop, and I left it on the bed." Now we know she is describing a container for money and the connection is made between "perk" and "purse."

Another way to clarify a comment you don't understand is by a technique called indirect repair (Sabat, 2001). In this method, the listener clarifies a comment, not through direct questioning but by listening to the intent of the statement and repeating one's interpretation back to the person for confirmation. In many cases, the overall tone of the sentence carries more information than the exact words.

Word substitution can also occur as a receptive problem; in other words, what *you* say may be misinterpreted by the person with dementia. It can be difficult to tell if this is due to poor hearing or a processing problem, but the effect is the same.

> Once I was visiting a woman with dementia, accompanied by Anne, the nurse manager. The woman, now in her late 80s, had a beautiful photo taken of her as a young woman that sat on top of her television set. I pointed out the photo to Anne, who turned to the woman and said, "Wow, you were quite a 'dish'!" The woman looked alarmed and said, "Did you say I was a bitch?" We were able to quickly clarify the misunderstanding, and later we all chuckled at the embarrassing episode.

While this example is rather humorous, some misunderstandings can amplify paranoia or agitation and lead to more significant problems. It is always important to check for understanding if there is any question that what you said was not received correctly.

Third-Person Speech

Many people with later stages of dementia appear to be talking about another person, and it is difficult to ascertain who that person is. In many cases the person she is describing is actually herself, but language difficulties have changed the grammar. It is common for people with advanced dementia to say, "She had a nice dinner" or "She doesn't have any pain," referring to themselves. Sometimes these thoughts will be projected onto a doll or stuffed animal. "She is a good girl. She ate all her food and feels very happy today."

In some cases, third-person speech can be combined with word substitutions. A person might say, "She was upset because her mother scolded her." Is that some long-ago memory? It may actually be that she was recently spoken to in a belittling way by a relative or staff member, and this is how the description of the event came out. This highlights an important principle in deciphering altered speech: Be attuned to the emotional content of the words, even if they don't make sense on the surface.

> Ruth was in her 90s and had advanced dementia. It was very difficult to get her to focus her thoughts and answer questions. She tended to sit quietly, but when approached in conversation, she would respond with long periods of run-on speech, barely pausing to breathe. Her speech seemed to ramble and not be based in reality: "And my father loves me, and he always comes to see me, and she had a good time and was very happy, and her mother was there, and the sun is shining, and . . ." and so on.
>
> Even when answering a direct question, Ruth would then drift off into the run-on sentences again: "No, I don't have pain, and my mother was there, and she was happy, and . . ."
>
> Aside from the brief answers I was able to obtain, I learned that most of my insight into Ruth's condition from day to day came from the *emotional content* of her words, rather than their actual meaning. Most days, her words, as described above, were positive and happy, and she seemed to be otherwise relaxed. The staff learned that such speech was part of her condition and did not try to make her stop.
>
> On occasion, the imagery in her speech would shift: "and she was bad and her father was very angry and she couldn't go to school, and . . ." This was often a clue to some underlying emotional or physical distress. We didn't always find the exact trigger, but the insight helped us to intervene in ways that might calm her and make her more comfortable.
>
> Another clue I discovered over time was that when Ruth was content, her run-on speech would stop after you said good-bye and walked away. On her more troubled days, the speech would often linger even after I walked out of sight.
>
> Most important, her care partners came to realize that her pattern of speech was a function of her dementia and her new way of expressing herself. It was never viewed as a problem that needed to be corrected or medicated.

Confabulation

Confabulation refers to a process whereby a person fills in gaps in memory or speech with false information. This is common in people who have damage to the frontal lobes of the brain, and it is a classic hallmark of the alcohol-related dementia known as Korsakoff syndrome. (This has also been called Korsakoff psychosis because the substituted details can seem quite bizarre.) It is important to recognize this syndrome, because it differs from true delusions or hallucinations and usually does not cause emotional distress. It often serves to supply the person with a worldview that helps him feel more complete and unimpaired. Therefore, unnecessary use of antipsychotic medication can be avoided.

Emotional Amplification of Speech Problems

A person's emotional state can have significant effects on his ability to process and form coherent speech. Communication that is marginal under normal circumstances can become impossible during times of heightened anxiety. This can cause an episode of severe agitation or aggression to deteriorate further. Specific approaches for agitation and aggression will be discussed in later chapters. The basic principle with language problems, however, is to create as calm a space as possible for communication. Calm, measured speech by the care partner can be critical to helping defuse a crisis.

Even in day-to-day situations, creating a safe and relaxed environment can greatly improve communication with people who have language difficulties. It can feel disheartening to be unable to communicate one's needs. In the following case, this inability to communicate (combined with a recent move to the nursing home) caused severe depression, which was greatly helped by making a meaningful connection.

Robert's family described him as a "Renaissance man." He had had a long and varied career path, working as a photographer, architect, inventor, and independent businessman. He had, however, developed a progressive dementia with much difficulty expressing his thoughts. When Robert's wife could no longer care for him at home, he moved to St. John's Home. In spite of his severe word-finding difficulties, he remained quite alert to his surroundings. The loss of autonomy and familiarity that accompanied his move caused him to become despondent in his early weeks at St. John's.

I was asked to see Robert one Monday morning because he had been acting more depressed over the weekend and was making comments about wanting to die. At one point, he had managed to say the words "I will suicide," and so there was great consternation on the part of the staff.

When I approached Robert, he was sitting in a TV lounge that was rather crowded and overstimulating. He seemed a bit out of sorts, and when I greeted him and made a few initial conversational comments, he seemed unable to answer coherently. He started to speak but kept getting stuck, unable to find the right words to complete his thoughts.

After I moved him to a quiet, private space, he still had great difficulty with expression. I realized that his anxiety was getting in his way. I began by looking inward. Was I anxious too? I was certainly concerned about his prior comments, and I was pondering whether he might be suicidal. Would I be able to tell? Would I need to consult with our psychiatrist to decide what to do? How could we address the grief he was feeling from this upheaval in his life?

I decided that I needed to find a calm, centered place and share this with Robert. Taking a deep breath, I let the silence sit between us as I slowed my breathing and relaxed my facial expression. The result was a softer, calmer, more measured speech.

I started with some general conversation, trying not to move too quickly into difficult territory. He began to copy my demeanor and relaxed, even smiled a bit. Eventually I moved toward the subject at hand by saying that I had heard of some troubles he was having. He asked, "When?" I told him it was over the previous weekend, and he said, "That's right." What follows is a very close approximation of our conversation from that point. Note how I repeated his comments, occasionally rephrasing them for clarity and to confirm my own understanding.

AP: What happened?

Robert: Well ... my mother ... is somewhere above. I was thinking of trying to get together photos for the kids, and ... I was ... trying to put together ... for the "loans" ...

AP: You wanted to arrange, or frame, some photos?

Robert: Yes, that's exactly it.

AP: For yourself, or for the kids?

Robert: Well, that's exactly ... but I seem to ... Well, there are problems.

AP: I know a bit about what has happened to you recently. It must be hard being in a new place and not being able to be with your wife and family.

Robert: Yes, exactly. It is very hard, but I think it is not something that would be unusual.

AP: No, it's quite natural to feel sad about these changes.

Robert: Yes, it is. Did they tell you?

AP: Yes, in fact, the nurses were concerned that you were feeling that life was not worth living anymore.

Robert: *(quietly)* I did not know that they realized that.

> *AP:* I think you may have said something about wanting to end your life.
>
> *Robert:* Did I?
>
> *AP:* I believe so. Do you still feel that way?
>
> *Robert:* Well, no. I believe I feel better now.
>
> *AP:* I know it's hard not being home, but your medical condition is such that you need to be here right now. But we want to help you to do as much as you wish. We need you to tell us what you would like. You are still in control.
>
> *Robert:* Well, that's very kind of you. I imagine that it is something that is not always the case.
>
> *AP:* Yes, that can be true, especially when people have trouble speaking their mind. So we need you to let us know what you like so that you can stay in charge.
>
> *Robert:* *(brightening visibly)* Yes! Everyone needs to have that, don't they? It is so good of you to tell me that. Thank you.
>
> *AP:* You're very welcome. Would you be willing to have Mary, our psychiatric nurse, stop by to talk to you a bit more about your feelings?
>
> *Robert:* Okay, sure.

There are many lessons to be learned from this conversation. Robert is a highly intelligent man, and he has always had a desire for precision. Now he has extreme difficulty even finding the words to express simple thoughts. When he became upset, there was very little that he could say that the staff could comprehend, which magnified his feelings of helplessness and hopelessness. Even when I sat down with him, he initially struggled to speak.

The foregoing dialogue does not detail all of our initial "small talk." Even so, this brief excerpt shows that Robert's speech improved over the course of the conversation. His initial attempts to speak were too disjointed for me to accurately record and remember. If the entire interaction had been captured, it would be clear that he began with a great deal of hesitation, stammering, and getting "stuck." By the end, he was speaking with relative ease and using fairly complex and complete thoughts. It can also be seen that his words are less circuitous and more precise toward the end.

There are several things that enabled this improvement to occur. First, we moved to a quiet, safe spot for interaction. I began by centering myself and calming my own emotions, which had a positive effect. Then we started a general conversation, keeping things open-ended and sticking to "safe" topics until Robert appeared more relaxed. At that time, I began to move into the more difficult subject of his depression.

As an active listener, I tried to stay focused and look for the emotion and meaning behind his words. I checked his comments to be sure I understood them correctly, and he was very able to tell me when I was on the right track.

The dialogue also shows a technique called validation, in which I acknowledged his personal experience and emotions in an empathetic and nonjudgmental way to show that I understood how he was feeling. Finally, I spoke to the losses he had sustained, and promised to work with him to maximize his quality of life and to ensure that he was "still in control." This was very reassuring to him.

I closed by encouraging Robert to be proactive in sharing his feelings and desires with the staff, and I let him know that we were going to talk to him further about his depression and not just "sweep it under the rug." Although I didn't solve all of his problems, the encounter left Robert more relaxed, focused, and less despondent than when I had first approached him.

I will speak more about validation and active listening in the upcoming sections on agitation and aggression.

Reverting to a Prior Language

Many people who are foreign-born have learned English as a second language. As dementia progresses, there may be a tendency to revert back to the language of origin or to mix the two languages together.

Having an interpreter for foreign languages is crucial to understanding the needs of those who cannot speak English. There are a few caveats, however. The interpreter may need to translate words and expressions that are not exactly the same in each language. As a result, the interpreter will often substitute her own approximation of the translation, which may cloud the meaning of what was actually expressed. If the interpreter is a close friend or family member, there may be biases in how statements are translated. The interpreter might "clean up" the sentences to make the person sound less confused, or she may add her own spin on what she thinks her loved one is trying to say. This can create barriers to understanding. On top of this, the other types of language impairments we have examined (e.g., misnaming, confabulation) may also apply to the person's language of origin, which will make it even harder to interpret. Nevertheless, there is no substitute for trying to find out what a person needs in her own words, if possible. Engaging a person in her own language can have remarkable outcomes.

Anna was German by birth and immigrated to the United States as a young adult. In her adult years, she spoke English well, but as her Alzheimer's disease progressed, she gradually reverted back to her native tongue, and even while using that language she became increasingly difficult to understand. I saw her one day in her later stages of dementia. She was eating poorly, had lost a great deal of weight, and her responses were minimal and not understood by staff. The weight loss was interpreted as a failure to thrive, associated with the terminal stage of Alzheimer's.

I have some working knowledge of German, so I decided to greet her accordingly. I asked her how she was feeling and got little response. I then asked her, in German, if she had any pain, "Haben Sie Schmerzen?" To my surprise, she nodded her head emphatically. I asked her, "Wo?" ("Where?"), and she pointed to one of her back teeth. We sent her to the dentist, who extracted an abscessed tooth. After the gum healed, she began to eat more vigorously and regained all of the weight she had lost.

Tangential and "Nonsensical" Speech

Some of the most challenging people to understand are those whose speech easily wanders off topic, or who seem to have no coherent expressions. Even in the late stages of dementia, however, the principles already described can be applied and often lead to valuable insights. Let's review them once again.

First, create a space for conversation that is calm, quiet, and safe. Center yourself and project a relaxed, accepting demeanor. Speak slowly and carefully, and be sure the person can see and hear you. Be aware of any discomfort or anxiety that may further cloud his ability to engage. Observe the person's own demeanor and body language. What does it tell you about his current state of well-being? Listen to his tone of voice and try to see if the words used have any emotional content. Try to catch little bits and pieces that may carry important information. You can pursue these by repeating them back and watching for his response. If something comes through, rephrase the comment and ask if this is true.

Sabat (2001) advises us as follows:

> All too often, our attention can become hooked by the linguistic errors committed in the speech acts of [Alzheimer's] sufferers. However, if we look past them and search for the deeper, underlying meaning, which is often expressed through extra-linguistic communication such as tone of voice, facial expression, gesture, and the like, we can eventually enjoy at least some success. (p. 217)

Sabat tells of a woman whose daughter told him:

> [H]er mother would often wear on her face a very troubled, clenched expression. However, when the daughter asked repeatedly, "What's the matter?" her mother was unresponsive. I suggested that the daughter ask instead, "Are you upset?" and when she did so, her mother responded immediately and quite fully. (p. 217)

Elsewhere in his book, Sabat cautions us further on this point:

> It is very important that family members and other caregivers be extremely attentive to the person's use of words, to look past the surface structure, and to use the context of the conversation as a guide in the process of "translating" what the afflicted person is trying to say. Without such an approach, the person can easily and mistakenly be construed as, positioned as, being tremendously confused and then treated as if that were true. (p. 51)

At the far extreme are people whose language has totally deteriorated to incomprehensible sounds. Making a connection can be very challenging, especially if they appear to be distressed or if their utterances are loud. Sometimes the best approach is to let down your own guard and use their rhythms and patterns to find that connection.

Laura Beck, creator of the Eden at Home workshops, came to know the Eden Alternative because of the humanistic care her father received at an Eden Alternative nursing home in Texas, after other homes could not meet his needs. Her father was a military man, always steeped in tradition and decorum, and the changes he experienced were difficult for Laura to accept at times. She tells a particularly poignant story from a time late in her father's illness:

> One day, I paid my father a visit. In the advanced stages of Alzheimer's disease, he was long past simply forgetting my name. He no longer walked or spoke. Instead, he had a language all his own, composed of various sounds and frequently uttered at the top of his lungs.
>
> Fresh from his bath this particular morning, I found him napping in his room. He awoke suddenly, wild-eyed, wild-haired, singing a loud, rowdy chant of nonsensical syllables. This vision of him overwhelmed me. My first reaction when I laid eyes on him was to reject what I saw. This wasn't the father I once knew . . . and I wanted him back.
>
> I stepped out of the room, overwhelmed. I wanted to turn and go, but something stopped me. I asked myself what I was afraid

of. The answer was clear—I was afraid of this happening to me. Once I named my fear, I felt like maybe, just maybe, I could push through it.

So I went in, sat beside him, and took his hand while he sang. We connected with our eyes—eye contact was something I hadn't gotten from him in a very long time. I began to envy him as I watched him dance between the worlds. He was exploring places I couldn't begin to go . . .

I found I felt honored to share that moment with him, to play a part in his unhurried dance out of this world; to have witnessed his last steps a few months ago, and to have heard him utter my name for the last time almost three years previously.

Watching him, I did not see him as the victim of a debilitating disease, but rather as an inspired messenger. He was entirely in the moment—full of unfettered playfulness. How long had it been since I'd stopped to celebrate a moment so exuberantly?

So I joined in and chanted with him. . . . This was one of the most intense and delightful connections I had ever had in the history of my relationship with my father. His eyes met mine for the first time in years. Deeply moved, I thanked him for the wisdom he had offered me—a reminder to savor the precious gift of every moment. And I realized . . . had I succumbed to my fear, I would have missed it all. (Eden at Home trainer's syllabus, p. 36)

Thomas (2004) recalled a speaking engagement in Alaska when he referred to dementia as a "tragedy." He was approached after the talk by a native Alaskan, who told him that in the Inuit culture, dementia was seen as a gift.

She said that when an elder with dementia made reference to seeing and speaking with long-dead relatives, it was taken as proof that the elder had been gifted with the ability to have one foot in this world and one foot in the spirit world. (pp. 283–284)

Much of the sadness that surrounds caring for a loved one with dementia involves dealing with our own grief and losses, as well as those of our loved one. While these losses cannot be erased, making connections in the moment can provide islands of peace and loving engagement in an otherwise stormy period of life.

In his keynote address at Alzheimer's Disease International in 2009, Richard Taylor objected to the overuse of reminiscence in people with dementia, because it brought to mind what he had lost or forgotten: "I need you to love me for who I am, not who I was."

The Secret Garden and the Spark of Life

Several nurses have jokingly accused me of hallucinating, because I will sometimes visit a person with advanced dementia and report that they said something to me when they have not spoken to others in months. I don't think I do anything magical, but I try to create a presence that is mindful and accepting. While it may not always be enlightening, this approach occasionally unlocks what Verity and Lee (2008) call the "secret garden." People with advancing dementia respond to a depersonalizing environment by withdrawing behind a "mental wall":

> In behind the "wall" is a flourishing garden full of life and all of their spontaneous creativity is in there. . . . You will only be invited into the secret garden if you are a very special person. . . . Only the person with dementia holds the "key" to unlocking this door and only they can choose who receives the key. (p. 32)

In the Spark of Life program, which uses a facilitated club-type atmosphere to reengage people with severe dementia, Verity and Lee (2008) teach facilitation as a nine-step approach that centers around a "lead by following" process. The opening steps reflect what I have described— creating a warm, accepting demeanor, and facing a person on an equal level (or better yet, slightly below the person's eye level to give him a position of slight superiority, since we are seeking permission to enter his world). The key is to make an emotional bond, a connection of spirits that allows access to whatever the person is still able to share.

The facilitator then looks for any spontaneous utterances and repeats or builds upon what is heard to try to draw out more. Each new expression can be followed by the facilitator in a technique that gradually draws out more and more interaction, sometimes with impressive results.

The first Spark of Life demonstration video profiles Cecil, a gentleman with Parkinson's disease and dementia, who was almost not included in the session because it was felt he wouldn't respond. He had been unengaged and nonverbal for over a year. As the video powerfully shows, by the end of a 1-hour session, Cecil is speaking in progressively more coherent and complete sentences. He is telling stories about the Great War, singing "White Cliffs of Dover," and actually making clever puns. His eyes light up with the unmistakable spark that Verity and Lee describe, and he leaves the session a new man.

When Dementia Care Australia recently called Cecil's facility to check in on him, his nurses reported that, 2 years after the video was filmed, Cecil "is still firing on all cylinders." One wonders, given the advanced state of his disengagement, if Cecil would even be alive today, much less an active participant, had he not had this ongoing opportunity.

Hilary Lee, president of the Society for the Arts in Dementia Care in Perth, Australia, studied the Spark of Life program for her dissertation (Lee, 2007). She found several positive results, which were grouped into four themes: (1) reigniting the human essence, (2) developing a sense of creativity, (3) being in their shoes, and (4) enabling success.

The first theme was evidenced by findings of increased confidence, with improved social and communicative skills in the participants. There appeared to be improved memory, or at least enhanced ability to retrieve data previously thought lost. The second theme of developing creativity was reflected in an increased sense of connection with other people, and the ability to enhance their communication with music, humor, and retelling of life stories. "Being in their shoes" refers to changes among staff and family members as a result of the program. Both groups began to see the participants as people with potential to learn and grow. The need to individualize care was better recognized, and all expressed a desire to share this philosophy with other care settings. Finally, Lee was able to show that the facilitation training created a model for success and sustainability.

When language is severely impaired by advanced dementia, speech therapy often has limited effectiveness, though some people can use letter or picture boards to facilitate some communication. However, even when traditional methods to improve speech fail, there are still other avenues that can have dramatic results.

Arts and Creativity: Back Doors to Communication

When traditional approaches fail, it is time to look for other ways to enter the secret garden. Enhancing positive emotions, stimulating the senses, and harnessing arts and creativity have all emerged as successful approaches to connecting with people with dementia. An experience at St. John's drove this point home for me.

> Annie had severe Alzheimer's disease. From the time she first came to St. John's Home to live, she had great difficulty speaking. Even when she arrived, she had a severe stuttering speech and could only occasionally produce a brief reply to a question.

In the years that followed, Annie lost all of her coherent speech. She continued to engage people with her eyes—she always smiled when I stopped by to see her—but whenever she tried to speak, all she could manage was a stuttering "Ba-ba-ba-ba." Annie's care partners learned to interpret many of her needs by her demeanor and the tone of voice she used when she stuttered. Often a rising tone of voice indicated a need to have her incontinence pads changed, for example. She was calm when she was comfortable, but she had not said anything comprehensible in years.

One day I was seeing Annie for a routine visit. I brought her back to the quiet space of her bedroom and used all of my best tricks to try to get her to talk. I engaged her at eye level, spoke slowly and clearly, smiled warmly, and received a warm smile in return. I gave her questions that could be answered with one word, with a "yes" or "no," with head nodding, and I used hand gestures to try to get a response. No luck. She would open her mouth to reply, but "Ba-ba-ba-ba" was all she could say.

I checked her heart and lungs and after a few more attempts to converse, I wheeled her back to the lounge. There was little activity there, but spotting a CD player on a nearby table, I asked Annie if she would like to hear some music. Her eyes brightened. I chose a Glenn Miller CD and the first song was "In the Mood." Annie broke into a broad smile, so instead of rushing off, I took her hands and "chair-danced" with her. She began laughing uproariously and tried to sing along with a tone-deaf "La-la-la-la." When the song ended, I told her it was nice to see her and that I had to go now. Annie looked at me, and without hesitation she said, "Thank you for coming to see me." I almost fainted!

What had happened to "unlock" Annie's brain? Was it the music or the outburst of happy emotion? Was it endorphins? Repressed memories triggered by the music of a bygone era? Increased circulation from swinging her arms, laughing, and singing? Whatever the case, I had momentarily opened a "back door" to her speech center that bypassed the doorway that had been closed by her dementia.

The stories of Annie and Cecil show that there are reserves in the brains of people with dementia—untapped areas that can sometimes be opened with the right approach. While traditional conversation encounters the same blocked passages, these alternative paths likely find their way through connections with other parts of the brain—those that deal with music, art, emotion, or sensory stimulation.

Stories similar to these (and Freda's story in Chapter 7) have been reported by people who use massage, therapeutic touch, art therapy, pets, and many other types of sensory stimulation or creativity. There are a multitude of connections throughout the brain, creating a multitude of potential back doors for people whose speech has been affected by dementia or other neurological diseases. As a result, many sensory modalities have been found to enhance engagement and communication and reawaken lost skills.

In 1998, Anne Basting developed TimeSlips, a program that uses creative storytelling to tap into the latent skills of people with dementia. After a great deal of frustration with reminiscence activities, Basting reports that she presented a picture to a group of people with dementia and asked if they could make up a story about it. Working sequentially and collaboratively, they were able to engage in creating a narrative for 40 minutes, accompanied by song and laughter. From this experience, TimeSlips was born. Basting (2003) reported that the interaction of memory and creativity in this social environment was important in preserving a sense of self. By nonjudgmentally tapping into imagination and using a facilitative style, the creative ability thought to be lost in people with dementia can resurface.

A study of the TimeSlips program in 10 nursing homes (Fritsch et al., 2009) showed increased alertness and engagement in the people living in the homes that participated, compared to people in 10 comparison homes. There were also more frequent social interactions, staff–elder interactions, and a more positive view of those with dementia by the staff members of the participating homes.

Many forms of the creative arts can be used to unlock retained abilities or even discover new ones in people with dementia who had never pursued the arts previously. Gottlieb-Tanaka, Lee, and Graf (2008) developed and validated a Creative-Expressive Abilities Assessment Tool, which can identify expressive abilities, monitor them over time, and compare the merits of various creative arts approaches.

Music, art, photographs, tastes and smells, movement and dance, stroking a pet, or holding a baby—all have been used to trigger such awakenings. Even the sensory experience and mindfulness of therapeutic touch or a massage can accomplish this effect.

Saving Face

One final important concept in communicating with people who have memory problems is the process of saving face. People who are aware of gaps in their memory can become very frustrated when pressed to remember details that they can no longer easily retrieve. This can be quite obvious when standardized memory tests are administered. Having to answer 30 cognitive questions in one session can be taxing to people who are repeatedly drawing blanks. It can make them feel confused and stupid. It can also provoke an angry outburst or a refusal to continue with the evaluation.

This difficulty plays out in a more subtle manner in normal conversations as well. Therefore, a seemingly harmless question such as, "What did you have for lunch today?" or "Was your daughter in to visit over the weekend?" may provoke anxiety or anger. With practice, care partners can learn to converse while subtly helping the person to fill in the memory gaps: "I hear you had lasagna for lunch. That must have been tasty." This technique can be used in reminiscence. Instead of saying, "Do you remember what we did for our 25th anniversary trip?" (just imagine the embarrassment of not remembering one's own 25th anniversary), one can say, "I was remembering our 25th anniversary trip to Washington, D.C. The cherry blossoms were so beautiful and we got to tour the White House."

Diana Friel McGowin (1993) shared her experience this way:

> Asking if I could remember a particular event was demeaning, whether I could remember or not. I felt much more comfortable when [my husband] simply recounted an event, as it left the door open for me to either listen to this "new" old memory or to join in his remembrance. . . . I was experiencing a mental breakthrough! From now on, I must concentrate on what I have, not what I've lost. (p. 98)

Taylor (2007) adds, "Please accentuate the positive with my recollections. Don't lie if I'm not accurate, but don't try to make me remember exactly like you do" (p. 155).

It is important to remember the subtle effect of how we phrase comments to people with dementia. As outlined in Chapter 5, the biomedical model places the problem with the people who have dementia, which can be a barrier to deeper insights into their unmet needs. Rephrasing comments in a way that enables people with dementia to help you understand them can empower them and improve their efforts to communicate. "There is a difference between saying, 'You're not being clear' and 'I'm having trouble understanding what you're trying to tell me'" (Sabat, 2001, p. 38).

This "face saving" technique is also helpful in social situations, where memory loss and executive dysfunction can lead to embarrassment in public places. One of my coworkers, Sharlene Freeman, told me the story of a friend who has Alzheimer's and how his wife helps him when they go out to dinner with friends:

> She knows that the menu choices are overwhelming to him, so she says, "Are you going to order the chicken, like you usually do?" Instead of reminding him that he forgot to open his napkin on his lap, she will say, "Since I'm unfolding my napkin, I'll just do yours for you as well."
>
> On the way out of the restaurant, there are some steps to negotiate, so she says to her husband, "Would you please take my arm, so that I don't fall?"

By filling in the gaps in memory and social graces, Sharlene's friend has found a way to keep her husband socially engaged, while avoiding potentially embarrassing situations that could discourage both of them from wanting to socialize in the future. Her comments also keep her husband feeling useful and empowered. In this way, he is able to avoid the isolation that can occur when people with dementia are shielded from social gatherings.

Eden Alternative board member Sarah Rowan told me that she had a small card printed up that said "Thank you for understanding my loved one has Alzheimer's." She would quietly pass these cards to employees they encountered in stores, restaurants, and other public places. She found "an amazing outpouring of compassion" from people as a result.

Now that we have changed our view of the person with dementia and honed all of our interpersonal skills, it is time to apply this paradigm to the common situations where expressions of need might otherwise lead to another medication prescription. The following chapters address several specific scenarios through "experiential eyes."

CHAPTER 11

"I Know You're My Friend"

General Advice for Anxiety and Agitation

Now THAT WE HAVE DISCUSSED basic interpersonal approaches, we will turn our attention to approaching people with various expressions of need. I will discuss specific scenarios in later chapters, but the information in this chapter can be applied in general to any person who appears to be in distress.

Any time a new sign of distress occurs, care partners should speak directly to the person whenever possible. The answer may lend important clues to a triggering event or an unmet need; at best, you might get a direct explanation that is easily addressed. If a simple answer is not forthcoming, it is incumbent upon the care partners to meet and discuss what happened. This meeting should include anyone with intimate knowledge of the person and of the specific episode. The group should apply their experiential eyes to facilitate a better understanding of what they have seen.

Repetitive episodes of distress should be carefully monitored, as this will help provide important clues to the cause and point to an effective response. There are many tools for doing this. Some, like dementia care mapping (designed by Kitwood's Bradford Dementia Group), can be very informative but are complex and require extensive training and documentation to use effectively. This training is not currently available in the United States, but a text by Innes (2003) gives a review of the process.

Such tools can be very useful, and I recommend that the reader investigate them further. However, it is beyond the scope of this book to describe them in detail; we will instead concentrate on basic approaches that can be applied without extensive training.

Dementia experts use a rich language to describe the process of investigating behavioral expressions. Rader and Tornquist (1995) refer to four roles that care partners must adopt: the magician, the detective, the carpenter, and the jester.

The magician is the person who is able to put herself inside the head of the person with dementia. Using role-play, imagination, and other types of "magical" thinking, she seeks clues to what caused the person to become distressed. The detective sorts through all of the available information about the distress, including the time of day and other factors, to try to discover a possible trigger. The carpenter then builds a care plan to address the issue and hopefully remedy the distress. And the jester is a reminder that, in this difficult and demanding work, humor is often a valuable asset, both in working with people who live with dementia and with other partners in care.

Kuhn and Verity (2008) refer to the enlightened care partner as an artist, "a person whose work shows exceptional creativity or skill" (p. 16). The artist of dementia care uses the tools of empathy, love, understanding, respect, playfulness, and encouragement to create "an attitude of positive intention" (p. 17).

In keeping with the theme of this book, I will use the experiential model as our central theme in describing how to help people in distress. However, because people with dementia are often older and have other medical conditions, it is also important to look at the interplay between medical illness and behavioral symptoms.

I will break our approach into three sections. The first section will outline a basic medical evaluation of people with behavioral expressions. (We will start here, although medical illness is not the most common cause of anxiety or agitation, and a medical workup is usually not needed.)

Next I will describe an environmental audit that follows our experiential model. Finally, the chapter concludes with further advice for interpersonal interactions with a person in distress.

Medical Review

Even though we are aiming to "demedicalize" the care environment, behavioral expressions can sometimes have medical causes. What are the situations when this is the case, and how do we proceed? I will give you my personal opinions, based on my own clinical experience. Keep in mind, however, that all medical opinions leave room for discussion and individualized approaches. The Spanish golfer Seve Ballesteros once said, "I don't trust doctors. They are like golfers. Every one has a different answer to your problem." While this is true to some extent, the following guidelines will help answer the vast majority of your medical questions.

The most important times to consider a medical evaluation are whenever a new or different symptom appears, or if distress appears in someone who is newly under your care and is not well known to you. Remember to look at the big picture. All of us have daily fluctuations in our mood, and people with dementia are no exception. Many care professionals are quick to look for medical problems and give medication at the first sign of distress, or when people seem to be a bit short-tempered. I often find myself reminding care partners that everyone has the right to have a bad day once in a while. Therefore, it is best to step back and look at a larger time frame rather than an individual event. Look for trends that occur over several days, or for an expression that is totally uncharacteristic for the person in question. Once you have confirmed a significant change, the medical approach should look at three possible causes: medication side effects, infections, and other medical illnesses.

Medications

It goes without saying that any medical evaluation should start with a physical exam. The other absolute should be a review of the medication list. The onset of a behavioral expression after starting a new drug or changing the dose of an existing medication should make one very suspicious; however, even when drugs and dosages have been stable, they are worth a look.

There are thousands of medications, each with a laundry list of potential side effects. Let's make it simpler. We are concerned about pills that can do the following: (1) affect the brain, causing lethargy, anxiety, restlessness, or confusion; (2) affect the ability to move; (3)

affect sleep; (4) affect bowel and bladder function; (5) cause an allergic reaction; or (6) cause a chemical imbalance or organ damage.

Drugs That Affect the Brain

The first drugs to review are those that cause sedation as part of their primary action. This includes minor tranquilizers, sleeping pills, and antipsychotic medications. These drugs are a common culprit, although they are less likely to be the cause if the dose has been stable for many months. Even with a stable dose, however, these drugs can occasionally cause confusion, because people's brains and other organs change over time.

Antidepressant medications can also cause sedation or confusion in some people, as can antiseizure medications (remember Joanie's and Julia's stories). Medications for Parkinson's disease can often lead to confusion, even hallucinations, in people with or without dementia.

The most likely drug offenders are any pills that have anticholinergic effects, meaning that they decrease the levels of the chemical acetylcholine in the body. This is the chemical that is primarily affected in the brains of people with Alzheimer's disease, so drugs that block this can make the symptoms worse.

There are a multitude of drugs that can have anticholinergic effects. I always remember the major groups by calling them the "anti's": antipsychotics, antidepressants, antiseizure medicines, and anti-Parkinson's drugs have already been mentioned. Two other major groups are antihistamines and antispasmodics.

The older brands of antihistamines are the most likely to cause confusion. Some of them are still found in cold and allergy remedies, but they are also commonly sold as over-the-counter sleep aids. Here is a rule of thumb for both prescription and nonprescription medications: Anything that you take to help you sleep can potentially sedate or confuse you. (This even applies to so-called natural remedies. If it helps you fall asleep, it is affecting your alertness.)

Antispasmodic drugs are used widely these days. There are three main reasons for their use: overactive bladder, irritable bowel syndrome, and muscle spasms. As we saw in Chapter 2, bladder relaxants can have subtle effects on cognition, even when the user has no known dementia. The medications used for irritable bowel syndrome are very similar to the bladder drugs in composition and effect.

Muscle relaxants usually produce very little benefit in older people, relative to their risk for sedation and confusion. I almost never prescribe them to older adults. Even in a person with dementia, a narcotic pain killer is usually safer and more effective than a muscle relaxant.

Narcotics can occasionally be a problem but usually do not cause confusion or behavioral symptoms if dosed carefully. Many people who claim to be "allergic" to narcotics simply reacted to having too much medication given too quickly. When the occasional person has a true allergy, changing to a different brand often solves the problem.

Beyond these major groups, there are many more drugs that can potentially cause confusion or agitation, from blood pressure medications to over-the-counter arthritis pills. Even the drugs that are prescribed to slow the effects of dementia have been known to occasionally cause confusion or agitation. Once again, always review the medication list and keep a high index of suspicion, especially if a person is on several medications. If you find a drug that is likely to be the culprit, you have the option to either reduce the dose or stop the pill completely. Your medical professional can help decide the best approach for each situation.

Drugs That Affect Mobility

The largest category here is the group of antipsychotic drugs, which can cause a Parkinson's-like stiffness and slowness of movement. This can increase the risk of falls, and it may promote incontinence if one can no longer reach the bathroom quickly. In addition, many of the sedating drugs discussed above can cause gait imbalance or incoordination, leading to falls, increased anxiety, and agitation.

Drugs That Affect One's Sleep

In addition to the sedating effects of many pills, there are also drugs that may *decrease* sleep. The most common stimulant is not a pill—it is caffeine. Evening caffeine use should always be eliminated when one is caring for people with sleep disturbances. Many other drugs can cause sleeplessness, including some antidepressants, as well as the attention deficit/hyperactivity disorder drugs that are sometimes used for depression in older adults.

Drugs That Affect Bowel and Bladder Function

Drugs that slow bladder activity can cause confusion and even urinary retention, leading to agitation. Those that increase bladder function or have a diuretic effect can cause incontinence and nighttime awakening. Similarly, too much of a bowel laxative can be distressing, especially in a person with limited mobility. Many drugs can cause constipation or stool impaction, particularly narcotics and pills with anticholinergic effects.

Allergic Reactions

In addition to the side effects just discussed, some people have true allergies to medications. These reactions can cause anxiety due to severe itching or hives. Such symptoms may be felt even if there is no obvious rash. Many allergies, though not all, occur within days after starting a new medication. Antibiotics are by far the biggest culprits.

Drugs That Cause Chemical Imbalances or Organ Damage

Any upset in the body's chemical balance can cause anxiety or confusion as well. One common cause is a change in the level of sodium in the blood. Low levels can be caused by many medications, especially diuretics, certain blood pressure medications, and some antidepressants. Rarely, a drug may cause a high sodium level as well. Drugs that affect kidney, liver, or thyroid function may also produce confusion or anxiety.

Infections

Infections are a well-known cause of confusion in older adults, even those without a diagnosis of dementia. The delirium that accompanies infection often appears as a decrease in alertness, but anxiety, agitation, and even hallucinations may occur. Several possible sites of infection should be considered, but the topic of bladder infections deserves more discussion here.

We spent many years reminding professional care staff to think of bladder infections whenever people with dementia became more confused. I believe that we have learned this lesson a bit too well and are now overtreating people. The topic of urinary tract infection (UTI) is very complicated, especially when it involves people who live in nursing homes. Here is a summary of take-home points:

Many older people, especially those in nursing homes, have bacteria in their urine but are not infected.

Many older people, especially those in nursing homes, have white blood cells in their urine but are not infected.

Therefore, *a positive urine analysis or culture alone does not mean infection.* There must be other signs and symptoms to justify treatment with antibiotics. These may include fever, painful urination, new or worsening incontinence, or a significant change in alertness or behavior.

Unfortunately, many people who have only a mild fluctuation in their mood or behavior will have a urine specimen sent, and if there is any sign of bacteria, they are put on antibiotics, even though there is a high likelihood that infection is not the problem. This can be dangerous, not only by increasing the risk of an allergic reaction to the antibiotic but also by increasing the risk of the serious bowel infection *Clostridium difficile*, which can result from antibiotic use.

So how do we decide if a person really has a UTI? It can be very tricky. If there is an unexplained fever, pain, or other change in urination, then a positive urine culture can point the way to careful antibiotic use. If all you see is a behavioral change, it is less clear. In this instance, I would recommend that care partners confirm that this is indeed a significant change and not just a minor fluctuation. I would move more quickly to check the urine of someone who is somnolent, as opposed to someone who is anxious—they are not only more likely to be infected, but also adequate fluid intake becomes a more pressing issue in people who are less alert.

If a person has agitation without any other symptoms, wait for the urine culture to be completed. This will allow another 48 hours to observe the person. If the new symptoms persist and the urine culture looks infected, a trial of antibiotics may be warranted. *However, it is important to observe whether the behavioral symptoms improve as a result of the treatment.* If they continue to fluctuate on and off after several days' treatment, then there was probably another reason for the symptom. If it appears that a particular behavioral symptom was not caused by an infection, there is no need to keep checking the urine during future episodes unless they are accompanied by other symptoms.

Finally a word about hallucinations: I have seen rare episodes of hallucinations in people with infections. One woman at St. John's Home had two or three episodes of bladder infection, and each time it happened she saw chickens running around the lounge. The chickens disappeared after a few days of antibiotics.

Amusing anecdotes aside, however, visual hallucinations are not very common with such infections, and this should not be your first concern if true hallucinations appear. We will cover hallucinations in more detail in Chapter 13.

Other types of infection usually have accompanying symptoms that point the way to the diagnosis. Rarely, a person might have pneumonia without any outward symptoms, but unless a fever is present or the physical exam suggests an abnormality, I would not recommend routine x-rays in someone with a behavioral change.

Other Medical Illnesses

Many other medical illnesses can cause changes in alertness or behavioral symptoms. The list is long, but there are a few to keep in mind. The number one concern is always pain, from any source. Always look for pain, just as you would check the blood pressure or temperature. Chemical imbalances mentioned previously can also result from underlying illness. Changes in sodium and calcium levels are particularly likely to affect the brain. So can abnormalities in liver or kidney function, an abnormal sugar level, thyroid or parathyroid disease, and cancer. Even a heart attack or congestive heart failure can look like an attack of anxiety or agitation. It also goes without saying that a stroke or other brain process is likely to cause changes in alertness or behavioral symptoms. Usually there are other signs to guide you.

The Medical Evaluation

How far do we go in searching for a medical cause for a behavioral expression? I believe that the majority of these are not due to medical illness, with one important exception: *If a person becomes lethargic or somnolent, a medical illness or drug side effect is highly likely and should be carefully ruled out.* For those who are not less alert but have other behavioral changes, the foregoing considerations apply but are less likely to be the cause than environmental factors.

For a basic medical workup, always do a physical exam and look at the medication list. Beyond that, a basic blood profile will look at the electrolytes, sugar level, and kidney function, and a blood cell count may point to anemia or infection. A thyroid test should be considered if it hasn't recently been checked. Beyond that, I would let the symptoms, exam results, and past medical history dictate the ordering of any other tests.

Environmental Audit

The majority of people who have generalized anxiety or agitation will not have an acute medical problem. Although we are working to transform the overall care environment for people with dementia, there are specific factors in the environment we can review that may trigger a behavior change.

As mentioned earlier, pain and discomfort should always be considered. This may be made worse by the type of chair a person is using or her position in the chair. People with arthritis or spinal curvatures often do not tolerate a straight-backed chair. The seat may be too hard, or she may be leaning to one side. Even in the ideal seat, anyone can become uncomfortable if left too long without a change in position. Frequent repositioning and walking, if the person is able, can help. This may also be a sign that more pain medication is needed.

In a large living environment, the room temperature that is best for some may not work for others. Always check to see if a person is too warm or too cold. This can usually be easily remedied by changing the thermostat or one's clothing.

Bowel and bladder needs should always be assessed. Distress can arise from several factors: urgency to urinate or defecate, feelings of fullness from constipation or urinary retention, discomfort from a catheter or as a result of an episode of incontinence. Annie, mentioned earlier, was unable to speak coherently, but her care partners came to recognize that when she became verbally agitated, it almost always signaled a bowel or bladder issue. Their intimate knowledge of her greatly facilitated her care and helped get her off the antipsychotic medication she was taking when she first moved in.

Hunger and thirst may be causes of behavioral expressions. Another environmental factor is lighting (see Chapter 6). Over- and understimulation are also frequent causes of distress. The former is often seen in nursing homes, where many people occupy a living area. The latter is prevalent in an isolated community setting but can also occur right in the middle of a busy nursing home lounge, if there is little or no direct engagement with the individual.

A large part of environmental overstimulation relates to noise. I am using the word *noise* to describe any unwanted sound, but it may not be recognized by others in the vicinity as being unwanted or unpleasant. We quickly become immune to the sounds in our environment, and we often don't appreciate the sensitivity of others to these same sounds. In the institutional environment, I have already described the myriad beeps, bangs, pagers, and intercoms that create a disturbing level of background noise. Even when these are eliminated, however, normal ambient sounds need to be audited as well. How are people conversing? Is their tone of voice warm and welcoming, or is it harried, shrill, or demanding? As one's ability to process words declines, these nonverbal components become more pronounced. Are many people speaking at once, or is there a quiet, respectful exchange of ideas?

The verbal dimension has even subtler components. The choice of words is also very important. A comment may contain language that upsets a person with dementia. This should not be surprising, since we have all had the experience of offending another person in daily conversation with a poor choice of words. As described in Chapter 9, infantilizing language can also be offensive, even to people with severe dementia.

One more comment on conversations: if they are barely audible, such as outside a person's room, they may be interpreted with suspicion or regarded as hallucinations (see Chapter 13).

Beyond the scope of speech and institutional noise, the rest of the spectrum of environmental sounds may also either soothe or disrupt a person's state of mind. Music, for example, is universally considered to be beneficial, but what if it is too loud? What if it is the wrong style of music for a person's taste? And what if it is heard at a time when one wants a quiet environment, such as at night? The same considerations apply to birds, television, children's laughter, or water fountains. It is important to know the individual in order to determine if the environmental ambience is a blessing or a burden.

Competing sounds are also problematic for many people with dementia and can lead to an inability to focus one's thoughts. Bryden (2005) relates that background noise

> will make me tired and confused, anxious, and even aggressive. . . . I wonder why so many day care centers and nursing homes have a TV, radio, and talking all happening at once? No wonder the people sitting there all look so blank! (p. 145)

Finally, as outlined in Chapter 7, activities can be helpful or harmful for people with behavioral expressions. The factors that most determine the outcome include the size of the group, the level of commotion, the degree of match or mismatch between the cognitive level of the individual and the activity being presented, the level of engagement with the activity, and the overall comfort of the individual at the time.

At times activities can be constructed that allow a person to express herself using her behavioral expression as an asset, rather than a failing. Stehman, Strachan, Glenner, Glenner, and Neubauer (1996) have created activities that can be useful in people with perseveration (the tendency to get "stuck" on a particular activity and repeat it over and over). The authors suggest such activities as painting an object that requires large areas to be covered by one color, winding balls of yarn, kneading dough, or folding linen. Some of the suggested activities, such as ironing or playing catch, may be a bit too complex for someone who is truly perseverating. Other activities may feel meaningless to even a person with advanced dementia, and could increase one's agitation. Nevertheless, this approach is a positive step in finding ways to reframe an expression, rather than simply seeing it as a problem.

As you review each individual's care environment, these guidelines should help you discover other environmental factors that may affect each person's experience.

Approaching a Person in Distress

General Approach

Having reviewed the medical and environmental components of anxiety and agitation, I will now turn to the critically important topic of approaching the person in distress. Once again, individuals are unique in terms of their experience, but the following guidelines are a good place to start for the initial interaction.

The first point to make is that *a person in distress has a reason to feel that way.* It may not be apparent to those around him, or it may seem trivial or unrealistic, but from that person's point of view, it is very real. The experiential approach starts with that assumption and explores solutions within that framework, rather than trying to impose a different reality on someone whose composure has been disrupted.

A person who sees her care partners as unsympathetic, confusing, or controlling may even strike out in frustration. Communication starts from the moment you approach another person. First impressions count. The best approach to a person in distress is by one person alone, with a calm, accepting demeanor. In the same vein, your tone of voice transmits as much information as the words you use. I have watched care partners try to calm agitated people with very appropriate words, but their tone of voice conveys distress and frustration, so their words have the opposite effect of what they intended.

Read the following statements aloud twice; first as you would if you are harried and frustrated with the individual you are talking to, then again with a calm, peaceful, reassuring tone of voice: "Mr. Smith, please sit back down in your chair. I know you are looking for your daughter. She is not here right now, but she will be in to visit at dinner time. Everything is okay." Imagine how these words can create a markedly different effect on a confused, distressed person, depending upon how they are spoken. When approaching a distressed person with dementia, care partners often find that the emotion they display returns to them twofold.

Jane Verity (2002) stresses the central importance of relationship in creating joy and fulfillment for people with advancing dementia. Here is some of her advice:

> When you approach a person with dementia, it is important to project kindness and love. This means a calm, soft, friendly voice. This means a genuine smile—the type that starts with the eyes and spreads across the face, not the "fake smile" that only involves the mouth. People with dementia can tell the difference every time.
>
> If you are having a bad day, it is important to try not to take that into the person's room with you, especially if they are anxious or agitated. You must be able to approach an agitated person with a calm, loving heart. If you can't do that on a given day, get someone else to approach them, because you will only make things worse!

The presence of two or more people may be threatening to a distressed person and should be avoided unless personal safety is a serious concern. Also, it tends to lead to more than one person speaking at once or giving conflicting instructions, which will compound the problem.

As discussed in Chapter 9, it is helpful to position yourself at or slightly below eye level. This means that if the person is seated or in bed, you should try to sit down. If your original plan was to bathe or dress someone, this may seem like a burdensome and counterproductive use of your precious time. After all, you can't perform these tasks very well from the seated position. Nevertheless, a few minutes of quiet, seated communication can greatly smooth the encounter and save a lot more time in the long run.

Even when one is speaking in a kind and compassionate manner, standing over a person in distress conveys an image of dominance and control, which can cancel out all of the good intentions. At the same time, be aware of issues of personal space, especially in people who may feel defensive or threatened. Getting too close without permission could cause the agitated person to lash out physically.

Speech should be calm, kind, soft, and slowly paced—not as one would speak to a child, but slow enough to allow time for processing and response, and to convey that you are not about to rush away. If the person is anxious, try to make your voice a bit more melodious; if agitated or angry, try to keep your voice more level.

Always begin by asking how the person is feeling and by validating the emotion you see. Go to her "place," and don't try to contradict or explain away what she is experiencing. Even if you think you can explain or solve her dilemma, it is often better just to listen and to reassure the person that she is safe.

Reorient or Not?

When a person with dementia develops an idea not based in our reality, the preceding question is often debated. Most would agree that a harsh rejoinder, like "You're 92 years old—your mother has been dead for years!" is counterproductive. However, many care partners try to use more gentle language to bring an anxious person with dementia back to the here and now.

There is often a fear that not doing this will lead to further decline in memory and orientation. I am not a strong advocate of reorientation, especially in the context of acute distress. When someone is very upset, it is a rare occasion when reorientation will have the desired calming effect. Telling someone who is distressed that his perception is incorrect tends to add to that distress.

Let's digress for a few minutes and use a bit of medieval history to give an example. In medieval Europe, the known world was mapped with east at the top of the page, instead of north. This was done in deference to the direction in which the Holy Land lay. Therefore, the map of the known world showed Europe to the left, North Africa to the right, and the Mediterranean (meaning "middle of the earth") running vertically down the center. Map readers would begin by orienting the map—placing it with the east on top. Later, as East Asia was explored and added to the top of the map, it became known as the Orient.

Let's imagine a gentleman from the Middle Ages who accidentally falls into a time warp and appears in our modern society. Even for a learned scholar, this would be an incredibly disorienting experience, encountering paved roadways, electric lights, automobiles, and metal "birds" flying overhead.

For purposes of this discussion, let's assume you speak a common language. You encounter this very agitated fellow and attempt to calm him. He repeatedly asks where his home is, so you pull out a map of the world. But this map is totally unfamiliar to him, especially the lands and seas that lie beyond his known world. If you know a bit about European history, you can find a map that shows Europe as it was known in medieval times. That's a bit better, but something is still bothering him. England is "standing up" instead of "lying down," and the Mediterranean Sea is doing the opposite. You then remember that maps were viewed differently in those days, and you rotate the map 90 degrees to the left. Now he can begin to recognize the landscape and you can show him where he has ended up. He is not particularly happy, but he is much calmer.

In this case, a person without dementia is put into a situation where he has no familiar wayfinding cues. The most successful approach starts with discovering his frame of reference, finding a landscape familiar to him, and leading him from there. So it is with dementia. By introducing ideas that conflict with a person's worldview, we intensify the psychic conflict he is feeling and leave him without a rock to stand on. Give him that rock, even if it is not the one we are on. Then find common *emotional* ground before making any attempt to move him off that rock.

Holden and Woods (1995) reported that the practice of "reality orientation" has been shown to improve performance on standardized cognitive tests; however, this did *not* produce any significant change in behavioral expressions, and the authors agree that when a person is confused and distressed, such an approach is best avoided.

In fact, the poor results seen when attempting to reorient people in distress led Naomi Feil to develop the technique of validation therapy, best described in *The Validation Breakthrough* (Feil and de Klerk-Rubin, 2002). Jones (1985) defines validation therapy simply as a technique used for communicating with disoriented people by validating and supporting their feelings "in whatever time and location is real to them" (p. 21).

While validation therapy requires special training to master, there are some basic techniques that all care partners can use in the setting of heightened distress. The first step is always to center yourself in order to be calm, nonjudgmental, and mindfully present. Next, describe the emotion you are seeing and try to identify with how it must feel: "You seem very sad. It must be hard to not have your daughter here with you." Allow the person space to expand upon those feelings, which may provide clues to approaches that might help her feel better.

Crying is an appropriate avenue for expressing grief. It can be uncomfortable to watch, but try not to suppress or discourage it. It can often have a calming effect to allow someone to "let it out."

When you have made a connection at the emotional level, the person will sense that you are in tune with her feelings. If she has reasonable verbal skills, she will likely be able to converse further with you in a more trusting manner. At this point, talking about the focus of her distress may be possible, and a practiced care partner can generally steer the topic in a way that becomes less emotional and more reminiscent.

An example of this might be as follows: start with validating comments ("I see how hard it is for you to be away from your home. No matter how nice people are, there's nothing like being in your own place, is there?"); then move to a less emotional plane ("Where is your house? What does it look like? What's your favorite room in the house?"), and so on. The actual exchange will be longer, but this shows in brief how one can connect with a person in distress, then lead her to a calmer place without having to reorient her or even solve her conflict.

When a measure of calm and connection has been achieved, the decision to introduce any further orienting information must be highly individualized. Its success will depend on the fragility of her calmness, her ability to hold new information, and the potential effect of introducing information that could have negative repercussions.

An example of the delicate nature of this interplay is the person whose wife has died in the past, who cannot retain that knowledge and continually asks for her. If he is upset about her absence, reminding him that she has died may exacerbate the situation: "When did this happen? How did she die? Why wasn't I told? Did they have the funeral without me?"

Even with validation and calming techniques, the decision to inform him of his bereavement must be individualized. Some people may be able to move to a place where they can process that death and connect with the supportive people around them for solace. Many people, however, will become distressed at the news, or perhaps at the fact that they did not remember the death, as if they have somehow dishonored their spouse by not holding that memory. In people with severe cognitive problems, it may be best to simply say, "Your wife isn't here right now, but she is safe," and leave it at that.

Mimi Bommelje, therapeutic recreation specialist at St. John's, recently recalled three such people she had cared for. These recollections show the spectrum of responses to such situations and highlight the need to know each person well and individualize one's approach.

Flora was asking for her "mother" one weekend, and a staff member told her that her mother was "in Heaven." This caused her to be severely distraught, because she had meant to ask for her daughter and thought she was being told that her daughter had died.

Vera would ask Mimi where her deceased husband was. Mimi would tell her, "He's not here, Vera," to which she would reply, "He's dead, isn't he?" Mimi would say, "Yes, I'm sorry," and Vera would cry a bit, but then say, "I knew it."

Willie's family asked that he not be told about his wife's death. The staff complied, but a couple of months later, he commented that a woman at the home looked "like my dead wife." This surprised Mimi, who said, "I hadn't noticed the resemblance, Willie. What reminded you of her?" He responded, "Well, it's really just her glasses on a chain. My wife wore them like that."

Mimi said, "You miss her," and Willie answered, "Every single day." Despite (or due to) his family's silence on the subject, Willie knew when his wife stopped coming to see him every day that she was gone.

The following story is another demonstration of the power of an empathic, person-directed approach to a person who has just remembered her mother's death:

Social worker Cathy Unsino told me a story concerning Jean, a registered nurse, now retired, who worked at a nursing home in Rochester, New York. She related an experience in which Jean showed her remarkable skill at relating to people with dementia, while modeling a successful approach to any severe emotional upset.

Cathy and Jean were walking through the nursing home on their way to a meeting when they passed a woman who was crying bitterly. Jean stopped and asked the woman what was wrong. "I just heard that my mother died," she replied.

In spite of the fact that this woman was about 90 years old, Jean never commented on the likelihood of this being true. Instead, she touched the woman gently and said, "Oh, I remember how I felt when my mother died. It just tore me up inside!" The woman nodded sympathetically.

Jean spent a few more minutes validating the woman's sense of loss. Then she said, "My, that's a beautiful sweater you're wearing! Is that color periwinkle or lilac?" The woman smiled and said, "My mother made it for me."

Once again, Jean did not challenge this unlikely statement. She stayed with the woman's view of reality and validated the positive aspect of her experience: "You must love her very much. That is so beautiful! Isn't it wonderful how your love is so deep!" The woman smiled and responded, "Yes."

After providing validation and redirection, Jean added one more very special touch: gratitude. She said to the woman, "This has been the most beautiful moment of my day. Thank you so much!" This left the woman calm, fulfilled, and with a sense of worth.

Jean later discovered that shortly before her outburst, the woman had said to a staff member, "I have to get home—my mother is waiting for me." The staff member had responded, "Your mother died 40 years ago."

Pearce (2007, p. 13) introduces another model for connecting with the person in distress, using the acronym *IF LOST*:

Intend a connection

Free yourself of opinions and judgments

Love

Open to being loved

Silence and the art of being with the person who has dementia

Thankfulness

With regard to silence and the art of being, Pearce comments: "Many care persons and professionals still ask, 'But what can we *do*?' I dare to suggest that *being with* the person who has dementia in a loving presence might be entirely what is needed in the moment" (p. 109).

Thankfulness may be less intuitive, but it is very important. Expressing gratitude for each interaction helps to seal the connection and validate the person's worth.

Keeping Your Cool

When people with dementia are very angry, they seem to have a knack for making comments that "push your buttons." They can even hurl personal or racial insults. This can be very upsetting to a well-meaning care partner, and reacting to this can cause the encounter to deteriorate.

When faced with this situation, the first thing to remember is that it is the confusion and distress speaking, not the person. He has a different view of the world around him and is feeling frightened or out of control of the situation. Maintaining this accepting attitude is not always easy in the face of hurtful comments, but it allows you to separate the person from his words and continue to interact with him in a caring manner.

When I was in medical training at the University of Rochester, Dr. Timothy Quill was my mentor for outpatient medicine. He is particularly skilled at navigating challenging interactions with patients. He used to advise that I "try to find at least one positive thing about each person which you like or admire, and hold onto that." He also used to say, "The more you disagree with someone, the harder you should try to feel what it is like to be in his shoes."

Pearce (2007) echoes the need to find "anything positive to connect with" (p. 30). She later adds:

> When I discover something I truly admire or like about the person with dementia, I get a key into my own state of loving. I can think about that aspect and let it fill my heart with admiration as I enter the room and greet her. When my heart is warm and positive, I greet her without agenda, prejudice, or anticipation. (p. 75)

The best approach to calming such a person needs to be individualized. Some people respond well to a validating comment ("You seem to be very angry. This must be frustrating for you."); however, others may just get annoyed with this approach ("Of course I'm angry, you idiot!").

Another approach is to look for a way to introduce a bit of choice into the situation, so that the person feels more in control. Offer to help him with his concern, and ask if he would like to sit for a minute, or go somewhere else to talk. This approach gives him some input, and it may also enable you to move a loud confrontation to a less public place.

Occasionally, a person may stand in the hallway in a very agitated state and may resist any attempts to move or redirect him. Recognize when this is the case and try to defuse the anger on the spot rather than forcibly leading him away. If this is unsuccessful, try to optimize the person's safety, then walk away and allow him a chance to cool down. Adding more people to the mix will usually make things worse.

Putting It All Together—An Example

In the Prologue, I mentioned during Simone's story that I was able to intercede in a very positive way during one of her biggest outbursts. I will describe that interaction in detail:

> I had been called by the nurse manager because Simone was very agitated one Friday afternoon. She was standing by a linen cart, angrily grabbing and rearranging washcloths and towels, and she struck out at anyone who tried to redirect her. When I saw her standing there with a furious expression on her face, roughly handling the linens, it was obvious that she would not easily be touched or moved.
>
> I donned a warm, affectionate smile and approached her with a hearty greeting, as I would any good friend or relative. She greeted me, but did not change her facial expression or activity. I stood close, but not too close for her comfort. I made no attempt to question or interfere with her activity; instead I conversed with her as she "worked."
>
> I began by asking how she was doing. Interestingly, she said she was "fine," as she scowled and worked furiously. I inquired about her family and she said she had not seen them recently. (She had no immediate family, and one of her nearest relatives had just had a baby and wasn't able to visit often. In fact, the less frequent visits could have contributed to Simone's increased distress.)
>
> I observed that she spoke to me as if I were a family member and she began to ask me how things were "down at the lake." Rather than correct her mistake, I latched on to this identity as a possible aid to communication. I told her everyone was fine, and that the family all sent their regards.
>
> This seemed to calm her slightly—there was a subtle softening of her expression, and her movements with the linen seemed a bit less violent. I continued to allow her to direct the conversation, answering her questions with very vague but reassuring comments about the family, and inserting my own family members when asked "how the kids are doing."
>
> At no time during this exchange did I attempt to get her to stop what she was doing. The normal tendency when seeing all of those clean linens being handled would be to steer her away, but she was not in a state of mind to allow that. Nevertheless, after about 5 minutes of casual conversation, she was connecting with me, speaking more calmly, and fingering the linens in a less purposeful manner.
>
> When I felt she looked calmer and less focused on rearranging

the linens, I followed one of her family queries by saying that I had some photos of the family down the hall in her room. Would she like to look at them? I was pleased when she readily agreed. She set down the towel in her hand and we walked together down the hall to her room. We sat on her bed and looked through a small photo album her family had left for her. She continued to become calmer with this reminiscence.

After several minutes of this activity, I asked Simone if she would like to hear some music. She said she would love to, so we walked to the dining room, which had a piano. I played a few old melodies, and we were soon joined by another gentleman and his daughter, who made several requests. I asked Simone if she had a favorite song, and she said, "Lara's Theme." When I played it, she had a look of complete serenity. After a few more songs, I left her smiling, with a hug and a promise to visit again soon.

Thanks to eBay, I was able to purchase a small music box that played "Lara's Theme," which brought her a bit of comfort in the days ahead.

Simone's respite was a brief one, and she ultimately had more serious problems, as I described in the Prologue. In fact, about 6 to 7 hours after the above interaction, she had another episode of agitation. Some of the staff felt that there was little to be learned from my approach because, after all, the agitation had just returned later. This is a common mistake care partners make.

Here's how I answered that comment: Suppose a person breaks her hip and has severe pain. You give her a pain pill and the pain gets better. But what happens in 6 hours? The pill wears off and the pain comes back. After all, her hip is broken! Does this mean that the pain pills are not worth giving? Of course not. The pills have a period of effectiveness. When that wears off, the dose must be repeated. It would be silly to think that a person with a broken hip could stay pain-free after a single dose.

An intervention for agitation is much the same. It is a single moment in time. My intervention left her calm and happy for several hours, but eventually her lack of connection to the environment around her caused her anxiety to increase once again. And like the person with a broken hip, she needed repeated "doses" of positive, validating interaction to produce lasting effects. By not having the resources to provide these in a consistent manner, we were unable to produce a lasting improvement in her overall experience.

But we need to take this one step further. The biomedical model views nonpharmacological interventions like doses of pills—discrete interactions superimposed upon the same old institutional environment. What is *really* needed in order to make a lasting impression of interventions like the one described is a transformed care environment that continually nurtures those who live and work there.

There is another important message here. The fact that I was able to engage one of our most challenging people at the height of her agitation and leave her relaxed and smiling for many hours shows that such interactions do indeed work. This is further proof that these interactions need to be woven into the fabric of everyday care. This underscores the importance of creating an environment where the elder is well known, and of creating interactions that boost self-esteem and individual meaning throughout the day.

Kuhn and Verity (2008) say it best:

> If you think of self-esteem as a bank account, your residents seek to keep a positive balance. . . . Whenever you or I succeed at something—no matter how small—and that success is acknowledged in a genuine way, our self-esteem account increases. However, the self-esteem account can be drawn down by negative experiences. . . . After awhile, your self-esteem account may drop so low that you don't wish to take a risk again. This is also true of people with dementia. . . . They may retreat into a private world where they feel safe and free of failure. (pp. 28–29)

A person with advanced dementia may not remember the names of her care partners or be able to recall the individual events of the day, but she will develop an internal sense of place, for better or worse, which will be built upon the number of positive or negative interactions she has experienced. My mother-in-law, who had severe Alzheimer's disease in her later years, once commented to my wife, "I don't know your name, but I know you're my friend." This, to put it simply, is our ultimate goal.

CHAPTER 12

"I Want to Go Home"

Approaches to Specific Scenarios

Now that we have reviewed a general approach to distress in people with dementia, this chapter will turn to some specific expressions that are commonly seen. As in Chapter 11, this chapter will look at medical, environmental, and interpersonal factors behind each situation, and then use the experiential model to craft some nonpharmacological solutions.

First, however, let's be sure we are ready to reframe our view of these expressions, and not just see them as problems to be managed. Rader and Tornquist (1995) state that "one of the first questions we need to ask is 'Whose problem is it?'" (p. 17).

Kuhn and Verity (2008) ask:

> Why can one person say or do something that does not bother you when another person who says or does the same thing really irritates you? Behavior is not a problem or difficult or challenging until you label it as such. (p. 55)

To Kuhn and Verity, the first step in bringing the "artist" in each of us to bear is self-awareness: "These situations often reveal how you feel about yourself, your relationships, your beliefs, your sense of humor, your sensitivity and your self-confidence" (p. 54). The authors add that this self-awareness is particularly helpful when a person's expressions are upsetting others:

> Because you are not consumed by negative emotions, you can devote your energy to . . . look for the meaning behind the challenging behavior and try to address the unmet need that is being expressed in an unpleasant way. (p. 55)

Bryden (2005) takes the concept a step further:

> This is called "challenging behaviour." Well I believe that this is "adaptive behaviour," where I am adapting to my care environment. I am pushing you when you want me to have a shower, or spitting out my food because I don't like it, or going to the toilet in the wrong place because I don't know where the toilet is, or walking into the wrong person's room because I don't know where my room is. Shower us or bathe us at a familiar time for us. Find out what food we like. Leave the toilet in clear view. If we can't read numbers anymore, why not mark our rooms with a distinctive sign. . . . If the care environ-ment is focused on the person and their needs, none of that so-called "challenging behaviour" needs to happen. (pp. 128–129)

Each of these authors is telling us that what we commonly view as a problem is often an expression of need in someone who may not be able to express that need in another way. Now that the challenge has been offered, let's look at some common scenarios.

Pacing and Wandering

When people with dementia start pacing or walking about, their activ-ity can appear to be purposeless and confused. By now, however, it should be clear that there are many other ways of looking at this. I will describe medical and environmental triggers, then move into the deeper realm of meaning.

From a medical standpoint, a primary trigger for restlessness is physical discomfort. Anyone who is unable to sit for long without pain will want to move about frequently. Another cause is restlessness related to the drugs themselves. Antipsychotic drugs can cause a severe motor restlessness called akathisia. While this classically occurs with older antipsychotic drugs, the newer brands have also been identified as a cause, as have many of the newer antidepressants.

In his memoir of prison life, *In the Belly of the Beast*, convicted murderer Jack Henry Abbott wrote of his experiences with this disorder:

> These drugs, in this family, do not calm or sedate the nerves. They attack. They attack from so deep inside you, you cannot locate the source of the pain. . . . The muscles of your jawbone go berserk, so that you bite the inside of your mouth and your jaw locks and the pain throbs. For *hours* every day this will occur. Your spinal column stiffens so that you can hardly move your head or your neck. . . . You ache with restlessness, so you feel you have to walk, to pace. (Abbott, 1981, pp. 35–36)

The following account by "Jennifer," a biomedical physicist, typifies the many similar experiences reported from akathisia:

> All I can say is that I hope none of you have experienced [akathisia] and never will—*it is pure hell.* You get so restless—it's like this inner turmoil compels you to move, like you're eating yourself up alive inside. . . . Sitting still was impossible—sometimes I absolutely had to pace around, other times it was okay to sit as long as I was tapping my feet, playing with a pencil, bouncing my knee, twirling my hair, or all at once. (2008 Web post, used with permission)

Increased violence in schizophrenics has been attributed to akathisia (Sachdev, 1995). No direct study has shown this in people with dementia, but it should be considered as a possible outcome. The symptoms can be improved by removal of the drug, addition of the beta blocker drug propranolol, or an anticholinergic drug (which of course can further confuse the person).

Akathisia may be missed if the restlessness is mostly internal and muscle symptoms are less apparent (Breggin, 1997; Hirose, 2003). Therefore, practitioners may mistake akathisia for persistent anxiety or aggressiveness and *increase* the drug, further compounding the problem.

Many drugs have a stimulant effect, which can cause pacing. These include caffeine, cold preparations, some herbal remedies, and some antidepressant medications. Any drug that has anticholinergic properties can cause a general feeling of restlessness, including the same drugs that treat akathisia.

Medications that cause the urge to urinate or defecate may bring about pacing. Similar urges stemming from underlying bowel and bladder disorders, like incontinence or infection, can have the same result.

Some other medical conditions that can cause pacing and restlessness are depression, neuropathies, skin disorders, and thyroid disease. The list of medical conditions is long and should be considered when such a symptom first appears.

Finally, the brain changes of dementia may lead to restless pacing. However, other causes should all be considered before simply concluding that the symptom is due solely to brain disease. Many aspects of one's environment can lead to pacing and wandering. Discomfort can arise from feeling too hot or too cold. Many people with dementia will get up and move rather than express their discomfort verbally.

The level of stimulation can have a similar effect. This could be either understimulation (leading one to look elsewhere for engagement) or overstimulation (leading one to try to escape the commotion). A third possibility is that the type of stimulation does not match a person's cognitive level, leading to frustration or boredom.

Experiencing an unfamiliar, institutional environment can make a person attempt to leave. Another trigger is the "end of shift" phenomenon, with the sight of care staff and visitors putting their coats on and heading for the door. A longstanding work history or prior lifestyle may lead to restlessness at a certain time of day.

I once cared for a gentleman in the nursing home who became restless and began pacing late each afternoon. This was attributed to "sundowning" behavior as a result of his dementia. However, his family mentioned that he had had a previous routine of walking his dog before dinner every day. A guided walk with a staff member each afternoon greatly calmed him, such that he was able to attend quietly the rest of the evening.

Holden and Woods (1995) remind us that we need to think of prior evening routines as well as daytime activities:

> Often at home, the evening is a time for change; the working day is over and these hours are used for relaxation and enjoyment, according to individual taste and circumstances . . . yet in care situations there often seems to be little difference. Many "odd" behaviours may have an explanation in relation to this. . . . It is accepted that activity is necessary during daylight hours, but it is also important that something different should happen in the evening. Apart from well-established habits, some activity in the early evening, followed by a more peaceful or routine activity, is thought necessary to evoke satisfactory sleep. (p. 131)

As always, the key is to know people's life stories, adapt the environment, and individualize the routines.

Even at home, people with dementia are often confined to a small living space, as their families are fearful of taking them outside. As a result, most get inadequate exercise, especially those who have a long history of being physically active. This lack of exercise can lead to poor sleep as well. Nighttime wandering can have many of the same medical and environmental causes. In addition, dementia can cause disorientation to time, disruption of the sleep–wake cycle, or an inability to separate dreams from reality. Each of these can lead to late-night activity. This can become a pattern that makes home-based care next to impossible for family members and often leads to sedative medication and all of its consequences.

The preceding discussion of environmental triggers touches on the relationship of *meaning* to the individual with dementia. Let's delve into this concept a bit further.

We have discussed the way our institutional approach to dementia can strip the care environment of meaning for the individual, and how important meaning is to well-being, even survival. Let's now replace the term *wandering* (which suggests an aimless activity) with *searching* or *exploring* (which suggests a sense of purpose). This lends new insights into the activity.

The experiential approach asks us to try to understand what a person may be searching for. In many cases, it is simply *home*—familiarity. In the nursing home, there is often very little that holds meaning for an individual other than a few possessions in her room. There is often nothing in the other living areas that "speaks" to her. Unfamiliar care partners who provide only superficial interactions also augment feelings of unfamiliarity. And an operational structure in which people come and go in a task-directed fashion (instead of stopping by to visit and connect, as we would in our own home) adds to the unfamiliarity and discomfort as well.

Nursing home workers are all familiar with people who rummage through others' rooms and hoard items they find. The experiential model tells us that such behavior may simply reflect a person's search to find objects of meaning in an environment that has little to offer. It is not enough to say, "She doesn't know that music box (or photo, or sweater, or jewelry) isn't hers because she's confused." An enlightened approach asks us to look carefully at those objects in an effort to find the underlying meaning of what she has taken. They may be symbolic of what is lacking in her world. Our experiential approach to pacing and wandering will start, as always, with a medical and environmental audit. These audits will directly point the way to many effective remedies.

Filling the void in meaning is more difficult work. As with other transformational processes, there are physical, operational, and interpersonal components to creating meaning. Bringing familiar objects into the care environment will help foster a sense of connection. Renovating a nursing home to create a "household" layout can also have a powerful effect.

> In 1999, I toured Fairport Baptist Home in Rochester, one of the first nursing homes in the country to remodel their living areas into "households" and remove the long hallways, nurses' stations, and medication carts. I was immediately struck by the different "feeling" of walking through this environment. I asked Reverend Garth Brokaw, Fairport's CEO, about his experience with people attempting to leave the building. He responded that there had been a marked decrease in this type of activity. His explanation: "When people live in a place that feels like home, they stop trying to leave."
>
> When Reverend Brokaw speaks about first moving to the household model, he tells people that he saw many behavioral symptoms improve "literally overnight."

The other aspect of the physical environment to consider is the creation of safe areas for exploration. Our experiential approach demands that we view such exploration not as a problem that must be eliminated, but as an activity that must be engaged while we look for other ways to fulfill the underlying need.

Creating a safe environment involves proper lighting, flooring, and footwear. It involves having a system to prevent unattended entry into stairwells, elevators, or the outdoors. There are many systems that help monitor the movements of people with dementia within their living environment. The less restrictive and institutional they are the better.

But there is a very important caveat here. The biomedical approach goes to great lengths to emphasize creating safe paths for wandering. While safety is important, it is not enough to modify only the physical environment. People wander because they seek meaning, identity, and connectedness with their surroundings. Most nursing homes never fulfill these basic needs; they merely provide a safe area for people to continue their frustrating and futile search!

I will not dwell upon the issue of physical restraints, except to say that I have not used one in my practice in over a decade. There are many resources available to help with restraint removal, especially since the Centers for Medicare and Medicaid Services have recently included this initiative in their "Ninth Scope of Work" project for U.S. nursing homes.

I recall a woman with dementia who was restrained with a "lap buddy" in her chair, which only worsened her agitation. At one point, this woman (whose dementia was classified as severe) said to a staff member, "Someone needs to explain to these people the psychological effects of restraining a human being!" Upon hearing about this, her social worker asked, "If a person can tell us that, doesn't that mean they should not be restrained?" My answer is, "Yes—even if she *can't* tell us." Another implication of avoiding restraints is that discussion will be needed about risk versus benefit in each situation. These conversations need to take into account the needs of the individual and maximize well-being wherever possible.

Of course, as this book has made clear, there is more to meaning and familiarity than the physical layout. Operationally and interpersonally, we must constantly create opportunities for autonomy and choice throughout the day. Life has meaning when we can exercise choice, weigh options, and create a rhythm of life that suits our personal style and needs. *This is no less true in people with advancing dementia.*

Creating this climate for autonomy can be challenging as a person's dementia becomes more advanced. There are several ways we can help the process along. The first is by never assuming that a person cannot give input into a decision until he is given an opportunity to try. We constantly position people with dementia, and pass judgment as to what they are or are not capable of deciding. Those who make the effort to make meaningful connections with such people are often pleasantly surprised at what they have to offer.

In looking at the causes of any behavioral expression, there are few as powerful as the feeling that you are in an environment that is beyond your control and constantly subject to the whims of others. We will look at this further in the next section on physical aggression.

Like meaning, creating familiarity goes beyond the physical structure and the furnishings. Even nursing homes that cannot afford to renovate can achieve dramatic results by fostering familiarity and trust through close, continuous relationships. Many people prefer not to travel alone to exotic locales, for example, because they value the familiarity of a close friend or relative as they explore new lands. In the same vein, I think that people with dementia can better navigate the unfamiliar landscapes created by their forgetfulness when they are surrounded by people with whom they have a meaningful relationship.

Social worker Cathy Unsino told me that she was once asked for advice about a man who constantly paced the halls of his nursing home, grunting loudly, with no coherent speech. She asked the staff, "What else do you know about him?" They knew little else, and had ascribed his behavior to severe dementia. After some research, they discovered that the gentleman had been the mayor of a small working-class town. He was very popular and was reelected many times, having served for 30 years. Cathy suggested that the staff tell him about their discovery and ask him what it was like to be mayor of that town. To their shock and delight, he began speaking coherently in great detail about his life.

The staff had finally made a meaningful connection with the gentleman and he responded. A staff member marveled that it was "the first time I talked to him like a person." The pacing and grunting stopped as the engagement continued.

The last aspect of creating meaning involves its incorporation into the rituals and rhythms of daily life. This was discussed in detail in Chapter 7.

One final comment about pacing: While medication may be used to treat pain, depression, or other symptoms that cause restlessness, the use of drugs specifically to keep a person from getting up and walking (so-called *chemical restraints*) should be avoided at all costs. Using sedation to prevent standing and walking creates a high degree of risk and, in my opinion, is indefensible.

Physical Aggression

Along with delusional symptoms (to be discussed later), physical aggression is the symptom most likely to lead practitioners to prescribe antipsychotics or other sedating medications. These episodes are particularly challenging because they present the potential for physical harm—to oneself or others—and often provide little time for reflection and investigation of one's underlying needs. Nevertheless, using our experiential toolkit, we will discover that such medication is far from inevitable.

There are three aspects of physical aggression that care partners need to address: dealing with aggression as it happens, investigating the cause, and employing approaches to minimize the risk of recurrence. Let's start, as we usually must, with tips for defusing the episode as it occurs.

When confronted with actual or threatened violence, I suggest you follow this sequence: provide safety for all, create space, restore calm, and then debrief.

Aggression can be directed toward family members, care staff, or other people living in the environment. Many of us can quickly move out of the way, but some cannot. A person whose mobility is impaired may be unable to get "out of the line of fire"; the same may apply to a care partner who is physically holding or supporting the person who becomes aggressive.

People in the vicinity who cannot walk should be moved to a safe location. If you are holding onto an aggressive person, find a way to help him into a fairly safe position and let go as quickly as possible. This cannot always be done delicately. It may be necessary, for example, to disengage and step away from a person even though you know him to be unsteady on his feet. If he is squeezing your arm, use your free hand to pry his fingers away. Keep your face and sensitive areas out of arm's length. Remove throwable objects from easy reach.

Once all people are physically safe from harm, it is best to have only one person interact with him. Ideally you should be the only person in sight, unless you have an extreme concern for your personal safety.

These first two steps in the sequence are often undertaken simultaneously. Thus you are creating physical space at the same time that you are removing yourself and others from harm. The other reason to create space is that many episodes of aggression are caused or exacerbated by crowding of personal space, which can make a person feel threatened.

Phair and Good (1998) emphasize that a person with dementia may repel care partners who enter the "intimate zone" of between 6 and 18 inches from another person. This space should not be entered without either "an invitation ('nurse, come and help me with my buttons') or an explanation ('I'm just going to brush your hair, Mrs. Jones')" (p. 75).

The third step, which has also likely begun at this point, is to use your voice and demeanor to try to restore calm. This can be extremely difficult if you feel surprised, angered, or frightened by the episode. It is essential to try, however, because failure to do so often results in failure to defuse the aggression.

As I mentioned in the previous chapter, a calm voice works best with aggression, but the voice should also have a firm, steady quality. Fear can underlie aggression, and even in the midst of an outburst directed at you, the person may find calm in your tone of quiet assuredness. This is very different from using an authoritative tone of voice. Feeling loss of control is a major component of aggression, and a voice that attempts to dictate behavior will likely meet with further resistance. Finding the right tone takes practice and is not always easy to master in the heat of the moment. You should adjust your tone as you observe the response you are getting.

As stated before, this is not usually a situation where a smiling face will help. In the experiential eyes of the person who is feeling threatened, a smile can look like a sneer and is often interpreted as mockery or making light of one's distress. In trying to be friendly, I have made this mistake on more than one occasion.

Because nonverbal signals are so important, the facial expression and body language will often trump the words that are spoken. If a stern face looks like a challenge and a smile looks like a sneer, then the best expression is often one that is placid, but also as expressionless as possible. Take the message out of your face and put it back into your words.

Your body language can also defeat the calming effect of your words. While keeping yourself safe, you must nevertheless remember the components of a good "face to face" approach: being at or below his eye level, using good eye contact, and trying to keep your posture relaxed and hands unclenched.

Just as an authoritative voice is counterproductive, the tender or "singsong" voice that can calm feelings of anxiety may magnify an angry outburst. To understand why, remember to go to his "place," his reality. In his world, there is a serious and imminent threat to his well-being, and such a tone of voice is inconsistent with the mood he is experiencing. These instances of emotional mismatch intensify distress in an environment that already feels confusing and threatening.

Now that you have set your facial expression, body language, and tone of voice, he is able to listen to what you say. You must choose your words carefully. According to the experiential approach you should not argue with or deny the reality of what he is feeling. If possible, validate his feelings, but try not to overdo it (e.g., "I know exactly how you feel."). You probably don't, and he knows that.

As you respond to his feelings, you move into the debriefing phase. You can use your validating comments to explore the reasons for his outburst and begin to search for a solution to his distress. For example, a validating statement ("It must be hard to feel like you're not in control of your life") may encourage him to expound upon that feeling and reveal what triggered it on this occasion. Once a calm dialogue is established, you might even ask, "What can we do to make things better for you?" He may now be focused enough to make specific requests that his care partners can try to fulfill in the future.

Remember that the person with dementia is always the best source for information about what he is experiencing, so use this interaction to glean as much insight as you can. Asking directly also sends a powerful message that his thoughts and feelings are important to those who are caring for him.

If these approaches do not have a calming effect, the best approach is to keep your words simple and few: "I'm sorry you're upset" or "I will talk to your nurse about this." If he says something that is highly offensive, he shouldn't be made to feel embarrassed, but it is perfectly acceptable to state that certain language is not acceptable to use with other people. If you are unable to calm him in any way, then it is time to maximize the safety of his surroundings, walk away, and allow him to calm himself.

Moving beyond the acute episode, it is time to review what happened and investigate possible causes that can be avoided in the future. From a medical standpoint, aggression due to medication is rare. However, as mentioned, akathisia has been known to cause violent outbursts. Delirium and other types of delusional disorders can also trigger aggressive acts.

There are other common medical causes, however, that are frequently overlooked. A recent study (Leonard, Tinetti, Allore, and Drickamer, 2006) of physical and verbal aggression in people with dementia found that depression was the most common cause. And while hallucinations were identified as a risk for aggression, an equal risk arose from constipation!

With aggression, it is critical to examine the care environment closely. While some episodes may appear to be unprovoked, in my experience there is usually a trigger. It may seem trivial, but keep in mind that dementia decreases a person's ability to cope with stress, tolerate commotion, or express his displeasure to those around him. I have found that many, if not most, episodes of aggression center on the loss of control over a person's surroundings. We have seen that our institutional approach to dementia robs people of control in all care settings. This lack of control leads to overwhelming feelings of frustration. This should come as no surprise, as it happens to all of us when we find ourselves in a similar situation. Some people are able to cope with this adversity; others suffer from depression and stress-related illness.

Dementia further impairs our coping ability. Those whose coping abilities are compromised will often respond to these feelings of frustration by lashing out. Most of the identified environmental triggers, such as excess commotion or infringement of personal space, feed into this loss of control and frustration. Much aggression occurs during personal care, when resistiveness and combativeness are common. In the task-driven institutional model of care, little attention is paid to the rhythm and needs of the person with dementia, because the demand for efficient completion of one's tasks takes priority. The natural tendency is to speed up the pace of care to resistant people, to "get it over with more quickly." This usually worsens the situation and is less efficient in the long run.

In spite of our desire to provide compassionate, high-quality care, we must acknowledge that we often do so purely from the standpoint of our own frame of reference, following our own priorities. We must broaden our view to better understand the perspective of the person for whom we are caring.

Cohen-Mansfield (2005) has shown that many incidents of physical aggression can be directly tied to the manner in which the person was approached by the care partner. It stands to reason, therefore, that those incidents could potentially be preventable without using medication. Cohen-Mansfield and Mintzer (2005) advocate for a new emphasis on nonpharmacological approaches, and they fault the current system for inadequate education and allocation of resources to provide individualized care, echoing the central theme of this book.

What else does this tell us about prevention of further episodes of aggression? It is all about autonomy and control. This requires consistent relationships with care partners who employ active listening. Active listening is an essential skill and one that is easy to learn, and yet it is underutilized in most care settings. It is the best way to empower another individual and give him meaningful input into the day-to-day decisions that affect him the most. Pearce (2007) reminds us that we generally don't give people enough time to express themselves because of our fix-it mentality:

> . . . the tendency to jump into problem-solving mode. This cuts off the person's expressions prematurely and denies his right to have a voice. As we bounce through our guesses about interventions, he can often feel invalidated or even more isolated. Sometimes he blossoms into full-blown rage or simply recoils into himself. (p. 141)

Sheafor and Horejsi (2006) recommend several steps to facilitate active listening. The listener needs to be "present" for the speaker, paying close attention to both the words and the feelings or other nonverbal signals being expressed. One should respond with a clear and engaged tone of voice. One's body language should also reflect interest and attention, to encourage the speaker to share openly.

The authors also suggest four specific techniques to facilitate understanding: (1) clarification—asking questions back to be sure you have understood properly, (2) paraphrasing—repeating the statement back in different words to help clarify that you understand the feelings expressed, (3) reflecting—taking factual statements and putting the underlying feelings into words for confirmation, and (4) summarization—putting all of the information together into a statement that sums up the ideas expressed, then asking for confirmation of what you have seen and heard (adapted from pp. 148–150).

Active listening also gives vital information for improving the experience of personal care and reducing the risk of altercations. There are various behavioral expressions that can arise during personal care, but I will use this section on aggression to outline some of the general approaches that can be tried.

If loss of control is a key factor, then care partners must look to restore autonomy to as much of the care experience as possible. This involves explaining each step that one is about to take, asking the individual to participate or direct the process as much as possible, and assuring that she is accepting of the proposed task before moving forward. We all instinctively know this, but it is amazing how often the institutional mindset causes us to skip over these important steps.

Let's begin with bathing. There is nothing inherently cruel about entering a room and saying, "Okay, Vincent, it's time for your shower." And yet this interaction immediately sets a potentially harmful tone by implying that Vincent has had no say in what is about to happen. The first step, then, is to find out when Vincent prefers to shower or if he prefers a bath instead. Once again, it seems almost too silly to write these words, and yet this happens all the time in care settings worldwide.

> Several years ago, I was doing medical rounds and my colleague, Dr. Michelle Carpenter-Bradley, was sitting in a nearby seat at the nurses' station. She suddenly began to laugh out loud, so I asked her what was so funny. She replied, "I was asked to evaluate a woman who is aggressive with care. I read her chart and this morning's note says, 'Resident was combative at 4 a.m. when taken for her shower.' Try giving me a shower at 4 a.m., and I'd be combative too!" Once again, institutional "efficiency" had trumped the individual's preference. The result was entirely predictable.

As mentioned previously, many care partners are reluctant to ask permission before performing a task. But even a refusal might give us insight into what makes the activity unpleasant. Most often, the person will be willing if the presentation and pace are respectful. It never hurts to inject little bits of autonomy into the process, even with people who have severe dementia. "Would you like me to wash your hands first or your face?" "Would you like to wash your own face?" Gentle cajoling can be useful: "I have the water nice and warm. Won't that feel nice on a cold morning?" Sharing personal stories and reminiscence can enhance the experience, as can soft lighting, music, and towel warmers. The result is *engagement*, not just body work.

Once again, for those who are predictably frightened or agitated by tubs *and* showers, Rader's bed-bath technique (Rader and Tornquist, 1995) is invaluable; the video *Bathing Without a Battle* (Barrick, Rader, Hoeffer, Sloane, and Biddle, 2001) is a must-see for anyone who cares for people with dementia. (The federal government sent a copy of this video to every nursing home in the country several years ago, yet I find that many care staff I talk to in my travels have never seen it and know nothing about the technique; hence my repetition of the method.)

Similar techniques can be applied to other aspects of care, such as dressing, dining, and trips to the toilet. For all care, I recommend the acronym *SEE*:

Slow down

Empower

Engage

I recently went to see a gentleman whose regular doctor was on vacation. I had never met him before, and the nurse informed me that he tended to stay in his room and that he had not allowed anyone to examine him in nearly a year. Personal care was accomplished with great difficulty, although his regular aides were able to make inroads on most days.

Even though I was only seeing him for a routine visit, I felt it would be useful to examine him, since it had been such a long time. I found him in bed, watching golf on television. A bit of casual conversation convinced me that the golf was just a distraction and that he was not particularly connected to the activity on the screen.

Looking for an inroad, I engaged him a bit and learned about his personal history. I asked him what he had done for a living. He replied, "I was a mechanic." I decided to try to use that information: "Most of the mechanics I've known have got very strong hand grips from using tools for so many years. Can I check your grips and see how strong you are?" He was only too happy to comply. I put out my fingers and let him squeeze them with his still-strong hands. Now we had made physical contact on his terms. I said, "Boy, you haven't lost your strength! I'll bet you have a strong heart too. Mind if I give it a listen?" I held up the bell of my stethoscope as I asked. Once again, he agreed. After complimenting the state of his heart, I moved through lungs, abdomen, and feet, then counted my blessings and bade him farewell, with a current physical exam to add to the record.

Most other identifiable causes for aggression can be managed by manipulating the environment. For example, if two people are constantly battling at the dinner table, they can sit separately. If noise and commotion are triggers, help the person to avoid such situations. Keep in mind that encroachment on anyone's personal space can feel threatening, as can care provided by more than one staff person at a time.

In some situations, a person's aggressiveness can be threatening enough that practitioners feel it is necessary to prescribe medication or even transfer the person to a hospital psychiatric ward or neurobehavioral unit for acute treatment. This may be necessary in extreme circumstances where immediate harm can otherwise result. There are some things to keep in mind, however.

Regarding medication, unless a person clearly has disorganized, psychotic thinking, any drug that is prescribed will reduce his aggression primarily through sedation. Resorting to this requires that we understand and accept that there may well be negative consequences, and that we are fairly sure that the potential benefit of such medication outweighs the risks. The care environment should then be investigated and modified so that the medication can be reduced as quickly and safely as possible.

It is also important to remember that an acute care hospital is not a "transformed" environment. The person's aggressiveness will be rapidly "controlled" through a combination of restraint and sedation. This means that even though the individual's aggression is halted, little else will be done to determine the underlying cause or help him to reintegrate successfully back into his living environment. Therefore, this approach is for true emergencies only and will not help you to provide a long-term solution.

Calling Out and Repetitive Speech

These are symptoms that many people try to reduce through medication, usually to little or no avail. As with other behavioral symptoms, sedation is a more likely outcome than true relaxation.

Addressing these verbal expressions requires a fundamental reexamination of our own feelings about what we are hearing. Once again, we tend to position the speech as being inappropriate, based on our "normal" frame of reference, without looking at other possibilities.

The experiential approach asks us to look for other reasons for repetitive speech besides the underlying brain disease alone. It also challenges us to look at our own attitudes about what does or does not constitute a "problem" (more on this in Chapter 14).

There are several experiential reasons why a person might have repetitive speech. The most basic is a lack of relationship, of connectedness to the surrounding environment. The person will therefore try to find connection by calling for a familiar person, usually a relative or trusted care partner who represents comfort and companionship to that person. So if a person repeatedly calls, "Mary, Mary," it is not enough to discover who Mary is. The key is not to supply Mary at all hours of the day, but to find out what qualities she represents and try to bring them to the living environment.

Once again, this is not a "quick-fix" solution. If there is no connectedness and meaning in the living environment, this cannot be solved in short order. But this once again illustrates the critical importance of transforming the care environment. This process must be ongoing or there will be no end to the string of future elders in your care who spend their days looking for "Mary."

If there is little response to calling out, the person may sometimes resort to grabbing at passers-by. Care partners are constantly trying to figure out, sometimes in exasperation, just what the person wants them to do, which brings them back to the paradigm of doing versus being. Pearce (2007) has some insight into this situation:

> It was not about her *getting* anything from me, or my *doing to* or *doing for* her. As Dr. Jean Baker Miller writes, "*it is about being in the flow of human connection, rather than out of it.*" (p. 10)

There are some ways you can start to address these needs immediately. Often, a few quiet moments sitting with such a person and holding her hand will produce a long period of calm. This is a case where sensory stimulation can be very calming, such as a hand massage or soft singing.

Pearce also suggests "four tools of 'being with'": (1) *touch*, gently creating relaxation and connection, (2) *observation* as a bridge to clues for causes of distress, (3) *encouraging the person's expressions*, and (4) *listening beyond the words.*

You can ask people what they need, but in my experience, people will rarely give you a specific request that can be easily met. Another option when someone is asking for a particular person is to say, "She's not here right now, but she is thinking of you." I once saw Joanne Rader approach a woman who was calling out, touch her gently on the shoulder, and say, "I'm right here." I don't see that as dishonest, because the woman was expressing a symbolic need and Joanne was fulfilling it.

Another type of repetitive speech is a more distressful cry, such as "Help, help." Once again, there is rarely a specific problem to be solved; rather, it is an expression of anxiety about being in an unfamiliar, possibly frightening, environment. A variation of this expression can be seen commonly in nursing homes among people who do not have dementia. St. John's CEO Charlie Runyon explained in a recent newspaper interview (Goldman, 2008): "Mrs. Jones is sitting there hitting her buzzer and says, 'Can you close those blinds?' Ten minutes later, 'Can you get me a sweater?' What Mrs. Jones *really* wants is companionship."

Another version of this is the repeated request to go to the bathroom. This happens frequently in nursing homes among people with and without dementia. Combine a weak bladder and a diuretic pill with limited mobility and you have a recipe for anxiety: "Is my aide nearby? What if she doesn't come right away when I have to go? I don't hold it well, and I don't want to soil myself. I had better go again now, just to be safe."

These physical sensations become magnified because of the institutional approach that keeps elders from being close to their care partners. The lack of close, trusting relationships, the task-oriented work schedule, and the physical size of the environment all contribute to a fear that help will not arrive in time.

Organizations that have transformed to Eden Alternative, Green House, or similar environments with close relationships report that these anxiety-related symptoms greatly decrease as a result. Once again, much of the answer comes back to transforming all aspects of the care environment.

One last type of repetitive speech I will discuss is the constant uttering of "nonsense" words or phrases. This can upset families and other care partners, who often rush to medication. Often, our investigation fails to give us any clue as to the significance of the words or phrases. What else can an experiential perspective tell us? If the environment feels foreign and frightening, then it follows that many people might use such speech as a form of "self-massage." If you bump your elbow, rubbing the area relieves some of the pain. What you are doing is creating a more pleasant sensation that competes for your brain's attention and pushes the pain to the background. Such is the effect of repetitive speech. In this setting, such words or sounds can have the same calming effect that people achieve by repeating a mantra or a religious catechism. We often use melodic songs or babblings to calm an upset child. If no one is there to help us, we can also do it to calm ourselves.

> Dr. Amy Mason took care of Lenore, a woman with advanced dementia. She had managed poorly both at home and in an assisted living setting, and had constant repetition of a nonsensical phrase that her care partners found very discomforting: "Casheladay, casheladay, casheladay," over and over. She had been medicated with a variety of potent drugs without success.
>
> One day, when Dr. Mason was visiting Lenore and attempting to examine her amid all of the vocalizations, she paused and spoke directly to Lenore, reflecting on her situation. Her comment went something like this:
>
> "Lenore, it must be scary to be in a place like this. You don't know anybody here, and you have no control over who is coming and going. I'll bet that saying those words over and over helps you relax a little bit."

Lenore suddenly paused in her constant speech, looked Dr. Mason squarely in the eyes, and emphatically said, "Yes." Then she resumed her vocalizations.

A humorous epilogue to the story is that some time after this conversation, Dr. Mason reported to me that she had a particularly frustrating day at work. At one point, sitting at her desk after finishing a difficult phone call, she just began loudly repeating Lenore's expression, several times over. "And you know what?" she said. "I felt better!"

By developing close relationships with people who have dementia, we may find other insights into this particular form of expression. My suggestion is to view it as that—a form of expression, rather than a behavioral problem—and see where that line of thinking takes you. Keep in mind that some vocalizations, especially those that are loud and accompanied by signs of distress, can be a result of physical discomfort. Don't forget to look for pain, incontinence, overstimulation, or other causes of distress.

I will close this section with a remarkable comment Cathy Unsino made to me about behavioral expressions: "People with Alzheimer's disease will help us make nursing homes more human by insisting that their humanity be affirmed."

Disinhibited Behavior

Certain forms of expression can be very distressing for loved ones and other care partners if they are disinhibited or frankly sexual in nature. Examples include lewd comments, inappropriate touching, public disrobing, or public urination. In the nursing home, there are sometimes people who will climb into another's bed, or two people with dementia who may "find each other" and share public displays of affection. Medication approaches have included various psychiatric drugs and hormonal treatments. All are fraught with problems. Is there a better way?

Let's look at a few specific expressions and examine them experientially. Lewd comments to people in the vicinity can cause staff, families, and other elders to be up in arms and demand that "something be done." The medical model of dementia tells us that damage to certain parts of the brain, especially the frontal lobes, can lead to such behavior, even in people who have never expressed themselves this way before.

There are other considerations to take into account, however. Much of the inappropriate language or touching that we see occurs during personal care—dressing, bathing, and helping to the toilet. Much of this care is provided by people who are not well known to the person with dementia. They are also likely to be younger and may be members of a different sex or ethnic background. Such intimate contact can be embarrassing to people with or without dementia. It may also be especially disempowering to have to rely on others for such activities. Men may feel less masculine if they have to depend on others to bathe or use the toilet. Such embarrassment can trigger comments meant to diffuse one's self-consciousness, and these can be expressed in sexual terms, as if to say, "I may no longer be able to walk or control my bowels, but I'm still a man, you know!"

So how can care partners help avoid this situation? One way is to keep care partners consistent, so that there is familiarity and trust. Another is to remember that providing care is a very personal experience and must be done with every attempt to preserve modesty and dignity. If someone's clothes are roughly removed and he is left to sit totally naked on a shower chair while being bathed, it is not surprising he would feel compelled to say something to dispel his embarrassment.

Another key point that is often forgotten is not to laugh at such comments. The person's comments may sound naturally funny, or it may be an effort to hide the care partner's own embarrassment. Regardless, laughing at such expressions will give a mixed message to the person with dementia that may actually reinforce the comment. It is not unkind to calmly and firmly state that a comment or touch is not appropriate.

Care partners always need to remember the power of touch. It can be very healing and soothing to people, but touch may also be misinterpreted. Always be aware of the effect your touch has on the recipient. The wrong choice of words may also embarrass or disempower a person with dementia, which in turn could lead to an outburst. It is critical that all care partners use a consistent approach to such expressions, in order to reinforce the proper conduct. At times, it will be best to use same-sex care partners for personal care.

Finally, be aware of cultural differences in one's style of approach or use of words. If there is a mismatch between the care partner and the person with dementia, there may be a misunderstanding.

From an experiential perspective, inappropriate or misdirected touch may arise from an environment that does not provide close relationships. It may also be triggered by the loss of daily contact with a spouse. Attention to the interpersonal aspects of the care environment, such as permanent staffing and affectionate, engaging care, is usually beneficial. Paradoxically, this behavior may also respond to an increase in more appropriate forms of physical contact, either during care or through modalities like massage, therapeutic touch, and aromatherapy.

Such modalities can provide a balm for anyone who is in need of more human connection. I will confess that I have occasionally ordered moisturizing creams twice as often as needed for people with dementia who are disengaged, merely to increase the frequency of hands-on contact.

Public disrobing should lead care partners to look at the comfort level of the environment. Often this reflects a need to cool down. Keep in mind that the "right" outfit in the morning may not remain comfortable as the day progresses. (Don't forget hot flashes, which can also be caused by medications.)

Disrobing may be due to itching from dry skin or other irritations. It may also be related to incontinence. Skin moisturizers or more frequent bathroom trips are often beneficial. One final possibility is that someone who is confused about the time of day or feeling sleepy is attempting to "get ready for bed."

As we investigate the possible causes of disrobing, there are some stopgap measures. A common one is to use a one-piece jumpsuit or clothing that fastens in the back and is harder to remove. However, keep in mind that if the cause is discomfort, these outfits might actually increase a person's frustration and distress. Always look for an underlying cause.

The "Sundown" Syndrome

The term *sundowning* refers to behavioral symptoms that worsen predictably in the late afternoon and early evening hours. This is commonly reported, though the exact cause is widely debated. Some people consider it a form of rhythmic delirium. Others propose changes in sleep patterns, effects of sleep apnea, or changes in the areas of the brain that affect the circadian rhythm—our biological clock.

There is no doubt that recognizing day–night cues is difficult for people who live in environments that don't allow much access to the outdoors, especially in climates with long, dark winter months. Adequate light also appears to increase serotonin, which can improve one's mood.

However, there are many considerations outside of brain function. Other aspects of the environment may cue certain responses. The sight of people leaving at the end of a shift in a nursing home, the act of sitting down to dinner, or seeing the evening news on television may trigger longstanding patterns.

We must also consider the care component of the late afternoon and early evening. How much of what we term *sundowning* is related to shift reports and lower staffing occurring at these times, resulting in fewer opportunities for elders to be active and engaged?

Once again, the experiential approach yields valuable insights. One proponent of this approach is social worker/consultant Cathy Unsino. Her first question to care partners struggling with challenging situations is to ask, "What do you know about him or her?" She will also suggest role-play whenever possible. She recently told me the following story, which shows a successful nondrug approach to a very disturbing situation:

Unsino was consulting for a nursing home and asked the staff to present the person they were "most concerned with." They told her about a gentleman I will call "Alex."

Alex was becoming agitated every night after dinner. Almost like clockwork, he began shouting loudly in a manner they considered to be confused. He would come to the nurses' station, open and slam drawers and throw objects around. Needless to say, he was disruptive and frightening to staff and elders alike.

As each episode occurred, staff had to forcibly remove him to his bedroom. He underwent psychiatric evaluation and medications were prescribed, to no avail. The diagnosis was "severe sundown syndrome, due to dementia."

Unsino began her session by asking, "What else do you know about Alex?" The staff reviewed his chart and everything else they had been told by his family. He was a former businessman, very successful, and traveled around the world in his profession. He was married, and his wife and children visited regularly and were very supportive. At this point, the staff had no more insights and felt this was "just sundowning."

Unsino suggested a role-play, to "get into his skin." This received a tepid response. Finally his evening nurse, who was very familiar with the episodes, volunteered to "play Alex." She sat at the dining room table and pretended to be Alex finishing his dinner.

The nurse then jumped up from the table, ran to the door, and began shouting his usual words, which had not been mentioned earlier: "I want a line! I want a line!"

Immediately, a look of realization came over the nurse's face and she whacked her forehead in exasperation: "He wants a phone line! He probably wants to call his wife!"

Because Alex was not able to use more specific language, he had failed to get his message across, and his agitated state caused his care partners to assume that what he was saying was nonsensical. In thinking about his long marriage to his wife, it soon became apparent that he might want to speak to her in the evening and say "Goodnight."

The next evening, as dinner drew to a close, the nurse approached Alex and asked if he would like to call his wife. Alex vigorously agreed, and was helped to do so.

In later conversations with staff, Alex's wife related that no matter where he traveled, Alex always used to call her each night. She now missed him most in the evenings, and she often lay awake at night worrying about how he was doing at the nursing home.

In spite of advancing dementia and language impairment, Alex continued to want to be a caregiver to his wife. Being "away from home," he wanted to speak to her and reassure her that he was okay.

Once the nightly routine was established, Alex's "sundowning" ceased, his medications were stopped, and his wife's insomnia was cured as well.

The moral of this story is that sundown syndrome, like other behavioral expressions, should not be painted with a broad brush when late-day expressions appear. In order to best discover the potential of unmet needs, you must individualize your approach and use your experiential eyes to help you understand what you are seeing.

If a medication had been found that successfully quieted Alex at night, he would not have been presented to Unsino as a person of concern, and a deeper examination of causes would never have been carried out. Think of the needs he and his wife had that would have been left unanswered.

"They're Poisoning the Food"

Nondrug Approaches to Paranoia, Hallucinations, and Delusions·

EVEN AMONG PRACTITIONERS who try to avoid giving antipsychotic medications to people with dementia, it is easy to "fall off the wagon" when people appear to have paranoia, hallucinations, or other delusions. However, like any other behavioral symptom, we should resist the knee-jerk response of prescribing pills and look more deeply into the nature of the problem.

There are three main points to consider when such symptoms appear: (1) whether the person truly is delusional, (2) whether this is an acute confusional state due to illness or a drug side effect, and (3) whether the transformed care environment can address the issue without medication. Even if you cannot totally eliminate medication use, it is surprising how often the nondrug approach can be successful.

Confirming the Diagnosis

Words like *paranoia*, *hallucinations*, and *delusions* are well defined by the American Psychiatric Association, but their use has crept into everyday language; as a result, many people use these terms rather loosely without making a careful diagnosis. Often there is a very good explanation for the symptoms we are seeing, if we use an experiential approach and don't rush to position the person as being confused or delusional simply because she has dementia.

Cohen-Mansfield (2003) explains that the psychotic symptoms of dementia are quite different from those of older people with schizophrenia and, therefore, one should not look at them the same way. She goes as far as to suggest that "it is time to abandon the word 'psychosis' from use with dementia patients" (p. 223). I agree that dropping this terminology would help us to look for other clues to the expressions we observe in the context of dementia. In my opinion, true psychotic symptoms are much rarer in people with dementia than most authors claim.

Bryden (2005) cautions that we should not be too quick to equate such expressions to those seen in psychotic illnesses. She suggests that this may be another form of adaptation to unfamiliar surroundings: "We misinterpret our environment, and try to make sense of it to restore our feelings of order" (p. 133).

In my educational sessions, I often invite participants to play a game I call "Don't Jump to Conclusions About Those Delusions." This is an activity that challenges people to think of alternative explanations for what is being reported. I will refer to some examples as we discuss each diagnosis.

Paranoia

Let's begin with paranoia. True paranoia is a condition in which one has feelings of persecution or jealousy that are *systematized*—that is, they are fairly fixed and recur over time. There is emotional upset that is consistent with the feelings expressed, and usually there are no hallucinations seen with this.

Many people are described by their care partners as paranoid when this is not truly the case. First of all, a single negative comment about someone does not qualify. Paranoia is fixed and recurrent, and these feelings are difficult to erase, even when one is presented with evidence to the contrary.

This is important in distinguishing true paranoia from forgetfulness. For example, a woman may leave her room to go to lunch and put her purse in a bedside table drawer for safekeeping. Upon returning to her room, she may forget this. If she doesn't see her purse when she returns, she may report that "someone stole my purse." Is this paranoia? It may be that simply showing her where she left the purse calms her.

Based on our discussion of the institutional model, it should come as no surprise that people who live in such environments might worry about theft. If an institution does not allow for people to develop close relationships with care partners or others in the home, a person with dementia will view her environment as a place full of strangers who come and go without boundaries. In a nation where many homeowners arm themselves against the possibility of theft, imagine how you would feel living in a place where you could not lock your door at night, where you had to share your living space and possibly even your sleeping space with people you didn't know.

Here is another classic statement: "They don't like me here." It sounds paranoid, especially if it is repeated over time and not shaken by care partners' reassurances. But is it really paranoia? Think about what happens to interpersonal relationships with an institutional approach to dementia. People are not asked for their input into daily decisions; they are often talked down to, or treated in a rough or impersonal manner. What would you think if you were treated this way, day in and day out?

Another common "delusion" is that one's spouse is unfaithful. Once again, the experiential approach shows this in a new light. Sabat (2001) relates the story of a man in a day program who harbored these feelings about his wife:

> One interpretation could focus on the fact that the man has [Alzheimer's] in the moderate to severe stages, his speech is incoherent, and we conclude that he has developed a delusion about his wife, because *we* know that his wife is consummately faithful. In this case his disease and its connotations form the conceptual scheme, the driving force, behind the interpretation. (p. 174)

Sabat then goes on to offer a different interpretation from the experiential point of view. The gentleman and his wife had been together constantly for years, but then she put him in a day program because she needed a respite. He was aware of his inability to help provide for her and, knowing that she was still "healthy, vibrant, intelligent, and attractive," it might seem reasonable to him that she craved the company of one more able than he. Sabat's approach, therefore, was not to dismiss the fear as a delusion, but to acknowledge that to this man it was very real, and to reassure him that it was not the case. And this only succeeded after he was able to spend several meetings "being" with him and gaining his trust.

Sabat quotes psychiatrist R. D. Laing (1965), who wrote: "One has to be able to orient oneself as a person in the other's scheme of things rather than only to see the other as an object in one's own world . . . without prejudging who is right and who is wrong" (p. 26).

Lastly, some people, young and old, view life with a personality that often has a paranoid "flavor." Have you ever encountered people who are always "victims"? Such people are quick to assign blame whenever things don't go their way. They tend to be distrustful of others and often are slow to accept any personal responsibility for bad decisions.

It is very important to recognize these longstanding "paranoid" personality traits in people with dementia, because they are not likely to be amenable to drug therapy and may need a behavioral therapy approach. Often, family and friends can confirm whether the observed behavior is a lifelong pattern or something new and different.

Hallucinations

Hallucination, like *paranoia*, is a word that gets overused and can be mistakenly applied. I would define a hallucination as a perception of something that has no objective evidence of existing. That "something" could be a voice or sound (auditory), a sight (visual), or something felt (sensory). Hallucinations of smell and taste are rare and more likely related to other neurological problems, like seizures, migraines, or tumors.

Because hallucinations manifest as abnormal sensory experiences, it is easy to confuse them with *misperceptions* caused by the changes that aging can produce on those sensory organs. Most people associate hallucinations with *seeing things*, so I'll start there.

If a person appears to have visual hallucinations, it is important to look for causes other than the person's dementia. It is likely that what he is experiencing is either a *false hallucination* (a misperception) or a true hallucination due to a medication effect or a medical illness. I will discuss drugs and medical illnesses in the second section on delirium.

The visual changes and disorders that can accompany aging can cause many misperceptions that are often mislabeled as hallucinations. In Chapter 6 we reviewed the need for increased light for older people, and the fact that most care environments do not provide adequate illumination. Therefore, shadows and poorly defined figures can produce misperceptions that look like hallucinations. The person who sees them may even say, "I think I'm hallucinating."

Thus it is not uncommon to hear that "there is someone outside my window" or "I think there's a man in my closet looking at me," particularly at night when lights are lowest. This can occur in people without dementia as well.

Fractured light and glare can also cause misperceptions. These may result from improper lighting or reflections from windows or mirrors. They may also result from structural eye problems, such as cataracts, "floaters," and detached retinas. People who have had strokes often lose sight in half of their visual field; as a result, people and objects positioned on the "blind" side may be misperceived.

Like visual hallucinations, those that are sensory often indicate a drug side effect. A classic example is someone using amphetamines or LSD who thinks he has bugs crawling all over him. Prescription medications can in rare instances cause a similar symptom, as can several common medical conditions, such as dry skin or neuropathy.

Auditory hallucinations are a hallmark of psychotic diseases such as schizophrenia. Even though textbooks may ascribe them to severe dementia, one should never view such a symptom as simply a natural consequence of the disease process. They are often misperceptions, or conditions that can be managed without drugs. They should always be investigated, not simply medicated.

The aging ear loses the high-pitched sounds first. This can reduce the clarity of consonants and make words sound indistinct. There may also be an overall loss of hearing, such that soft words may not be understood. It may be more difficult to discriminate sounds or locate them in one's environment.

When a person with dementia says, "I hear voices at night," it is often documented as a hallucination. But the hallucinations of schizophrenia are usually well-understood voices inside one's head, often making accusatory or threatening comments. Vague sounds in people with dementia are more likely a misperception.

Using the experiential approach, put yourself in the position of a person with dementia who has hearing loss. How would you interpret a voice coming over an intercom? How about soft conversation taking place outside your door? I recall a woman who was felt to have hallucinations because she was "hearing an orchestra play," but it only occurred in her room. It turned out that the woman in the next room, who was also hard of hearing, was playing her radio loudly enough for the music to filter through the wall.

As with paranoia, I will describe some environmental "cures" for these symptoms in the third part of this chapter.

Delusions

Delusions, like paranoia, are fixed ideas that are difficult to shake or explain away. Paranoia is a type of delusion, but there are many other types. One can have delusions of grandeur ("My son owns this place—I can have you fired, you know!"), of a sexual nature (a woman at our nursing home was convinced that she was pregnant, and that a staff member was the father), or of a variety of other bizarre ways of interpreting what the person is experiencing.

As a medical student, I once interviewed a gentleman with chronic schizophrenia whose thoughts were controlled by an evil computer named Harold Brown (who was President Carter's secretary of defense at the time). In my experience, these kinds of well-organized delusions are rarely seen in dementia. The kinds of delusions I have seen are less organized and often less fixed over time. As such, they require a different kind of analysis before we relegate a person to long-term antipsychotic therapy.

In order to illustrate the experiential approach to symptoms that sound delusional, let's look at five classic examples and try to find ways that a person's experience of his environment might trigger each of these thoughts. Such thoughts and statements often come about, not so much because of a true delusional disorder but through (1) defects in memory, (2) word-finding problems, (3) use of metaphor, (4) cultural and spiritual beliefs, or (5) very real experiences of personal care.

Defects in memory and word-finding problems often overlap, which can lead to a variety of misstatements. One example is the 90-year-old woman who smilingly tells you, "I had a nice day—my mother came to see me." Did she forget that it was her daughter who visited? Did she think her daughter was her mother? Did she forget she is 90 and that her parents died decades earlier? Did she simply slip and say "mother" by mistake, when she meant to say "daughter"? Any of these could be the case, and they often cause misstatements that can sound delusional.

Richard Taylor (2007) addresses this as follows:

> For instance, if I call you "Mom" or "Dad," I am probably not confusing you with my mom or dad. I know they are dead. I may be thinking

about the feelings and behaviors I associate with mom and dad. I miss those feelings; I need them. It's just that I so closely associate those feelings with my mom and dad that the words I use become interchangeable when I talk about them. I don't take the time or I can't or won't make the distinction between the people and the feelings. (p. 135)

"I had fun at work today." In this case, the statement could be the result of metaphor—what a particular activity symbolizes to the individual. A person in a nursing home may not have a job, but if she helps to sort papers, set the table, or fold washcloths, this may be the way she describes her activity. As we saw in the case of Sabat's "Mrs. D.," the act of socializing and lending friendship and support to those around you may bring the satisfaction of a job well done. And truthfully, is there any reason why a person should be made to believe otherwise?

Many years ago, I cared for a woman who told me on the day she moved into our nursing home that she saw Jesus and angels on a regular basis. In fact, her comments about these "visitations" had led to the family's decision to move her to a nursing home. Sometimes she would see them in her room or floating outside her window. Sometimes, it was merely a presence that reassured her and calmed her fears.

This was a very religious woman who now was developing moderate to severe dementia. Was this a delusion? Maybe. But maybe it was an expression of her deep and personal spirituality. (And, as our consulting psychiatrist once chided me, "How do you know they *aren't* there?"). Did I treat her with medication for this? No, never once during her life at the nursing home. I'll explain why in the third section.

In the nursing home or assisted living environment, it is not uncommon for a woman to claim that "I was raped." This causes great anxiety among staff and families. No one likes being accused of such a heinous act. We would never do such a thing! Therefore, it must be delusional, and, after doing the requisite exam to be sure it didn't really happen, we must treat it with medication. Or must we?

Using our experiential eyes, let's think about how the experience of personal care can be viewed by a person with dementia. If you do not recognize your care partners (or if they are constantly changing), they will be strangers to you. These strangers provide very personal contact while bathing people, inserting suppositories, applying lotions, or tending to catheters. If it is done in a rough manner, it can feel like a personal assault. Recall that Joanne Rader described the embarrassment of being bathed, even by people whom she knew and trusted. She told me that this led her to wonder how much worse it must be for a confused person who doesn't know her care partners.

One last example of a classic "delusion" is the statement that "they're poisoning the food." This certainly could be a delusional symptom, but maybe not. Many people who are reluctant to take their medications receive them crushed in applesauce, ice cream, or pudding, which they are encouraged to eat. The resultant bitter taste might very well cause a person with dementia to reach such a conclusion. If you hide a drug in food and don't tell the person about it, then you really are "poisoning" the food!

As this section illustrates, the experiential approach lends many clues to behavioral symptoms that are commonly labeled delusional or hallucinatory. The next section reviews the medical issues that must be considered when such symptoms appear.

Is It Delirium?

If we confirm that a psychotic symptom is not a misperception, nor due to other experiential factors, it is likely that this is not merely a symptom of dementia but may reflect an acute illness or medication side effect. In this case, it is more properly called delirium. As described in Chapter 11, there is a basic medical audit that will help investigate this further.

Any time such symptoms appear, medications should be at the top of one's list of possible culprits. The various drugs that have anticholinergic properties (see Chapter 11) are the most common causes, though many others can occasionally have this effect.

Begin by reviewing all medications. Focus first on recent additions or dose changes, then on the other "stable" drugs. Finally, think about potential interactions between drugs that could cause a toxic effect from an otherwise-safe dose. If there is any suspicion, try to reduce or stop one drug at a time so that you can more easily identify the offending agent. (The speed with which you do this depends on what type of drug is being reduced, how ill the person is, and how badly you think the person needed to be on the drug in the first place.)

I view visual and sensory hallucinations as most likely being due to a medication side effect. (An exception to this rule may be in people who have Lewy body dementia. In this disorder, vivid visual hallucinations are often described. However, the same investigative approaches should apply to this group, and nondrug approaches should always be considered, as these people are particularly sensitive to the side effects of antipsychotic medication.) When medications are ruled out, as discussed before, think of other medical illnesses causing delirium. Infections and strokes can occasionally cause hallucinations and delusions. Many other medical conditions can affect the brain as well, from lupus to thyroid disease.

Nonmedication Approaches

First and foremost is to create an environment where people with dementia have close, consistent care partners. This has many advantages. It creates the familiarity that promotes comfort, trust, and security in one's surroundings. It facilitates communication, as people with dementia will be more open to sharing their feelings, and care partners will be better able to understand them and find clues to their causes. Knowing a person well also enables care partners to recognize when a new and different symptom is occurring and to help brainstorm effective approaches that will suit the individual.

The importance of these relationships cannot be overstated. As long as an environment fails to provide this kind of care, one will never know for sure if the medications prescribed for such symptoms could have been avoided. The following story powerfully illustrates the many components of a successful care partnership:

The Story of Bertha and Missy

Melissa "Missy" Wormuth is a former nursing assistant who went back to school to become a licensed practical nurse. She was still relatively new to the field of nursing, but this story shows us that wisdom comprises much more than a title or length of time on the job.

Bertha has lived with us for nearly 5 years. At 93, she stands less than 5 feet tall and sports a black wig, which occasionally gets misaligned. She would be described as having advanced Alzheimer's disease.

Bertha has a very soft voice and always uses a polite and deferential tone, with head lowered, even if she is declining to follow a staff member's suggestion. It is not clear to me whether this results simply from a lifelong commitment to civility or from being raised in a time when people of color learned to keep their voices down when addressing authority figures. In any event, prior to the time of this story, she had never raised her voice or showed signs of any "behavioral symptom" other than an occasional polite "no thank you."

Bertha had been otherwise healthy and I had rarely examined her outside of my routine visits. I often say hello to her, but I doubt she remembers who I am. Missy, on the other hand, formed a strong bond with Bertha from the day she became her primary nurse. In spite of Bertha's reluctance to let me examine her at times, she always readily agreed when Missy came along.

On one summer visit, I found everything to be stable as usual. On the way back to the nurses' station, however, Missy related a story to me that shifted my own paradigm to a new level. Two weeks earlier, Missy had found Bertha in a highly agitated state, the likes of which she had never seen. Bertha was terrified that her son "Junior" was being attacked by vicious snakes. I think just about everyone would agree that she was experiencing a very frightening delusion.

Had I been called that day, I would have checked a urine culture, drawn some blood tests, and looked over her medication list. I also admit that I would likely have ordered at least one, if not several, doses of an antipsychotic drug for her intense distress. Most staff members would have called me for just that reason, but Missy did not.

Instead, Missy took Bertha to a quiet place away from the lounge and spent some time calming her and explaining that everyone was safe. She brought a telephone over and they called Junior, who reassured his mother that he was not in any danger. Then Missy got Bertha a snack and sat and engaged with her until she was sure the anxiety had passed. I first heard about this episode at my routine visit 2 weeks later, and it had not recurred.

It has been nearly 4 years since that day. Bertha has had significant progression of her dementia and is now receiving hospice care, but the snakes have not returned, and no antipsychotic drugs are being used.

In spite of my reluctance to use antipsychotics for agitation and anxiety, I had continued to treat frightening delusions in the traditional manner. This story opened my eyes to the possibility that even delusional symptoms could be addressed with a nonpharmacological approach.

There is a caveat to this story, however: If I or a different staff member had been the one to attempt this intervention, it may well have failed. Long before this symptom occurred, Missy had formed the close, trusting relationship that allowed her to successfully allay Bertha's fears. The importance of this bond cannot be overstated in the domain of caring for individuals with dementia.

Another critical point is that Sheila and Lynne, the nurse manager and nurse administrator who supervise Missy, have created a culture that allows her to be proactive in meeting her elders' needs in an empowered and individualized manner. No one criticized her for stepping outside her capacity or for not involving the doctor in the scenario from the start. She might not have been willing or able to try, had she worked elsewhere. This highlights the importance of operational transformation and empowerment in providing enlightened care.

There's an epilogue to this story. A few weeks later, it struck me that Bertha's frightening episode began in the television lounge. It also occurred to me that this was at a time when there were many advertisements for the new Samuel L. Jackson thriller *Snakes on a Plane*. The ads were pretty frightening—one more reason why random television programming may do more harm than good for people with advanced dementia.

Finally, I am struck by the knowledge that it would have been considered very fitting and proper for a practitioner to have given Bertha an antipsychotic drug, at least for a short time. No one in our biomedical model would question such a decision.

It is very sobering to think that many people would have accepted Bertha's episode as evidence of progression of her dementia, and felt that an antipsychotic drug was necessary due to her "worsening disease." Textbooks on dementia will tell you that such delusions are part of the "natural history" of advancing dementia. Bertha's dementia *has* progressed since then, but she remains delusion-free and drug-free. Many people are treated for weeks, months, even for life based on these single episodes. How many doses of a potentially harmful medication was Bertha spared over the past $3\frac{1}{2}$ years because of Missy's intervention?

What will be the next major advance in dementia—a cure for Alzheimer's? That would be wonderful, but I suspect that in the near future, the biggest breakthroughs will come to us, not from the research labs, but from the lessons we learn from the likes of Melissa (Missy) Wormuth, LPN.

Going to the Source

When worrisome symptoms occur, the first step in the investigation should be an attempt to hear these symptoms in detail, preferably from the person who experienced them. A face-to-face meeting can often bring new insights, unfiltered by the interpretations that can occur with word-of-mouth reports. Cohen-Mansfield (2003) reminds us that "in most cases, a physician prescribes antipsychotic medication on the basis of informant reports, without observation or direct contact with the older person" (p. 222). A personal visit can prevent potentially serious errors:

> Walter was a gentleman with Parkinson's disease and dementia who lived in a local nursing home. It was reported to me that he was hallucinating, having complained to the staff that bugs were crawling on the walls of his room. I had recently increased his Parkinson's medication, and it would have been a perfectly good assumption that this was the cause. I could easily have reduced the dose, or added an antipsychotic; I am sure there have been days when I would have done that. But it so happens that I chose to visit Walter in person that day. In doing so, I learned a valuable lesson.
>
> Even though he was forgetful, Walter had no problem repeating his complaint. In an effort to get more details I asked him to describe the insects to me. His eyes wandered as he mulled the question over; then pointing past me, he said, "Just like that one." I turned in time to see a cockroach scurry across the floor in the far corner of the room. It turned out that building renovations were driving the cockroaches out of the walls and into some of the bedrooms. Walter didn't need a medication change—he needed an exterminator!

Tracking Down a Cause

After eliminating the obvious, begin to look at the specifics of the symptom to determine what medical and environmental audits should be pursued. In the case of potential hallucinations, follow the sensory organ that is affected. If auditory, review causes of hearing loss and examine the sounds in the environment, especially those that we usually "tune out" but that could be very noticeable to a person with dementia. Does he hear a voice, music, or other sound? Is it distinct or vague? Are there specific words or phrases that can be recalled? Is there a particular location or time of day when this occurs?

For visual hallucinations, look at lighting levels and reflections in the room. Try to re-create the time of day and the person's vantage point. Be sure an eye exam is completed. And if there is still no good answer, look closely for medication effects or acute illness.

In addition to optimizing the amount of light, sound, and interaction in the environment, it is also important to preserve day/night cues as much as possible. Many people with dementia experience fractured sleep, and confusions of time and place can further complicate their perceptions.

Investigating abnormal sensations should involve a good skin examination and a thorough review of medications. Abnormal tastes may be due to medications or medical illness (e.g., acid reflux) but are not generally a sign of dementia. Abnormal odors, if not environmental, are likely due to problems in the mouth, nose, and sinuses, or a different neurological illness.

If the person's comments reflect paranoia or other delusions, start with a detailed description of what the person saw or heard and how it made her feel. Is it repeated over time? Does it occur in certain situations or with certain care partners? Is there an explanation for the person's experience that is acceptable to her?

Keep in mind that even a persistent feeling of persecution does not necessarily mean a need for medication. Often, it reflects inadequate communication, lack of close, trusting relationships, and other inadequacies of the care environment. These must always be addressed, or else no amount of medication will create a sense of ease.

> Nancy had advanced Alzheimer's disease and often made comments that had a paranoid flavor. A gentleman friend, John, came to visit her nearly daily, and she benefited greatly from his visits. At times, due to her attachment to John, his absence was very distressing to her, but she could never remember what time he was due for his visits, and she asked for him repeatedly.
>
> During a period of several days, she became quite distressed with delusional ideas that were directed at a nurse who was working per diem in her living area. Nancy was convinced that the nurse was having an affair with John and became very hostile and accusatory when the nurse was on duty.
>
> No one knows if a resemblance or past event made Nancy target this particular nurse; it never happened when anyone else was working. In this case the best solution, and the one we followed, was to reassign the nurse to another area where Nancy did not have to receive care from her. This took care of the delusion.

When discussing potential delusional symptoms, it is important not to challenge or argue with the person. The perception is very real to the person, and denying this will only heighten anxiety and resistiveness. If it appears that there is a simple explanation, one can attempt to reassure: "Here is your purse, in the bedside drawer. It wasn't stolen after all." But if that fails to satisfy a person's fears, there is little use in persisting along these lines.

It is critically important to take time to validate the distress a person is feeling, even if you see no clear reason for her distress. Care partners who skip this step often create a barrier between themselves and the person, who sees them as unsympathetic, unbelieving, or simply not an ally in helping relieve her distress.

When to Consider Medication

I believe that the vast majority of situations where medication needs to be considered are those of acute delirium, rather than symptoms arising purely from dementia. Even in delirium, however, the primary goal should be to *treat the underlying condition as safely and effectively as possible*. This means to reduce or replace any offending drugs, diagnose and treat infections, and stabilize other medical conditions. If this can be done without hospitalization, it will greatly reduce the risk of further complicating the delirium.

If it appears that the symptoms will not resolve quickly, the key to deciding about drug treatment lies in the nature of the symptom and the person's experience thereof. Keep in mind that adding another medication introduces another layer of potential side effects, so the benefit must outweigh the risk. Therefore, if the person's perception is not an unpleasant one, I would generally not prescribe medication.

In the case of the woman who had visions of Jesus and angels, these were recurrent visions that had a repetitive quality, but they were invariably comforting to her; her demeanor while describing them was relaxed, almost blissful. They also only appeared on occasion, often many days or weeks apart, so they did not suggest an acute medical problem. She lived at the home for over 2 years until her death, and these visions never increased in frequency nor did they degenerate into anything distressing.

On the other hand, delusions or hallucinations that are extremely frightening may require treatment, at least until the underlying disorder is addressed. Prolonged delirium can be toxic to brain cells, so it is important to reverse any underlying metabolic imbalance due to drugs or illness.

Another situation that may warrant treatment is one in which a delusional thought leads to potentially harmful behavior, such as refusing to eat and drink. Once again, there may be an experiential reason for this behavior, but if the person's health begins to suffer as a result, then a course of antipsychotic therapy may be warranted.

A final question to consider in deciding whether treatment is necessary is "whose problem is it?" Many abnormal thoughts and perceptions are more bothersome to loved ones or care partners than to the person himself. Here is how Cohen-Mansfield (2003) addresses this question:

> If caregivers, formal or informal, are disturbed by behavior that is very detached from reality, the intervention needs to target the caregivers and clarify what are appropriate and inappropriate goals of the intervention. Comfort and positive life experience are important goals, whereas experiencing reality in a way that matches that of caregivers is less important or relevant. (p. 221)

Summary

To summarize this complex chapter, I would recommend the following approach to any symptoms that look like hallucinations, delusions, or paranoia:

- See the person and discuss his perceptions with him, if at all possible.

- Hold a care partner session to brainstorm the problem. Use Rader and Tornquist's "magician" and "detective" approaches, role-play, and interview family members or other care partners for clues.

- Look for recurrence of symptoms over time. Try to avoid overreacting to the first episode of any symptom. Create and maintain a log of events to help find patterns or antecedents.

- Use the *experiential* approach. Always try to think like the person with dementia and see the environment through his eyes.

- Audit the living environment.

- Audit the interpersonal interactions within the environment.

- Audit the medications, do a medical examination (with special attention to the relevant sensory organs), and order laboratory tests as indicated.

- Remove offending drugs and/or treat acute medical illnesses.

- Try to reserve medication use for acute delirium with disturbing thoughts, or for chronic symptoms that are producing significant physical or psychological harm.

- If you must treat a disturbing delirium, this is one instance when you *should* choose an antipsychotic drug. Minor tranquilizers, antidepressants, and other psychiatric drugs are ineffective in this situation and potentially dangerous.

CHAPTER 14

"How Low Can You Go?"

Can We Achieve Drug-Free Care?

THE PRECEDING PAGES HAVE summarized the inadequacies and risks of the current model of care for people who live with dementia. We have reviewed some of the innovative schools of thought that are challenging the traditional model. Using these philosophies, we have crafted an *experiential* approach that can be applied to many common scenarios where potentially harmful drugs are often prescribed. The questions one might logically ask at this stage are: "Do these approaches really work?" and "Are they safer and more effective than our traditional approach?" All evidence to date suggests that the answer to both questions is "yes." But there are many gaps to be filled, and many professionals will find the current research evidence inconclusive and inadequate. There are several reasons for this.

First, the current research environment is such that much of the funding comes from vested interests, such as pharmaceutical companies. I would not expect a lot of support for nonpharmacological trials from this quarter.

Second, the principles of transformative models of care create a moral imperative that makes it difficult to follow the usual protocols. Is there ever going to be an ethical way to randomize subjects to receiving medication versus being treated with individuality, kindness, and respect? Kitwood (1997) addressed this question and concluded that "moral validity is not an empirical matter. It is merely a question of whether a form of care practice is logically consistent with an ethical stand that has already been given" (p. 100).

Third, the experiential approach outlined here relies heavily on a deep transformation of the care environment, including many interpersonal and attitudinal changes. This takes time and is very difficult to measure in limited trials.

Fourth, we have seen that current intervention studies do a poor job of measuring positive outcomes. Most of our "quality of life" scales are still rooted in biomedical thinking, and "well-being" has not been captured in the vast majority of research studies.

To this end, the Eden Alternative has convened a team to develop and validate a survey tool to measure the indices of well-being described by Fox et al. (2005): identity, growth, autonomy, security, connectedness, meaning, and joy. This tool (with separate versions designed for elders, their families, and care staff) is currently showing promise but may have limited use in people with more severe forms of dementia who cannot easily answer questions.

Lastly, the trend in nonpharmacological studies has been to follow the biomedical approach by testing only discrete interventions in an effort to measure a single variable (such as music therapy) that can be evaluated for benefit. But the experiential approach requires a wide range of transformative interventions happening concurrently. It would be futile to try to break them into separate parts for study because that is not the way the model is intended to operate.

Again, Kitwood (1997) supports this argument: "A better research strategy, I suggest, involves assessing the consequences of a pattern of care practice taken as a whole, without attempting to subdivide it minutely into separate variables." He goes on to say that even a "discrete" intervention, like music therapy, "involves many different types of interaction" (p. 100).

What I will offer, then, is a threefold response: some of the studies to date that support a transformative approach to care, my anecdotal practice experience, and the story of a trip to rural South Carolina.

Research Studies

Several studies connect transformative models of care with reduced medication use. Rovner, Steele, Shmuely, and Folstein (1996) studied

89 people with dementia in a nursing home. Half received usual care and the other half were enrolled in a program of activities while their care partners were educated on individualized care and medication guidelines. More than twice as many control subjects received antipsychotics or restraints, and the intervention group was 13 times more likely to participate in activities when offered.

Fossey et al. (2006) studied 12 nursing homes for people with dementia in the United Kingdom. The homes were randomized to receive either usual care or an educational program in person-centered care. After a year, antipsychotic use in the educated homes had dropped to 23%, versus 42% in the control homes, without any increase in agitated or disruptive behavior.

Ray et al. (1993) began a comprehensive educational program for doctors, nurses, and other nursing home staff. This program emphasized nonpharmacological approaches and reduction of antipsychotic medication. The educational program lasted for 4 months, and the homes were followed for an additional 6 months before and 3 months after the program. Antipsychotic drug use dropped 72% in the homes that received education, versus a 13% drop in those that did not. There was no worsening of behavioral expressions, even in those who had been off their medications for 3 months or longer.

Svarstad, Mount, and Bigelow (2001) showed a positive correlation between adoption of person-centered care practices and reductions in antipsychotic medications across 16 nursing homes in Wisconsin.

Equally important in transformational models is support and respect for the professional care staff in nursing homes. Cohen-Mansfield (2001) has shown that care partner support is critical to the success of the nonpharmacological approach.

Decades ago, Langer and Rodin (1976) constructed an elegant experiment on the effects of having control over one's environment in a nursing home population. The "choice" group was told that they had important input into their daily life and needs, and that they should let staff members know if there was anything they required. This group was also asked if they wanted to have a plant in their room, which they would care for by themselves. They were allowed to arrange their rooms as they liked and could choose which of two "movie nights" to attend.

In the comparison group, the *staff's* responsibility for the elders' well-being was emphasized. The residents were given a plant as a gift and told that the nurses would water it for them. They were told that their rooms were set up for them "to be as nice as they can be," without asking for any input from the residents as to the layout. They were each assigned to one of the "movie nights."

The group that was offered more choice and responsibility had several striking outcomes. First, they reported better health and happiness. Second, the nurses felt that 93% of the group's health had improved, versus 21% of the comparison group. The nurses rated the choice group as having greater levels of interpersonal activity and higher levels of alertness, and they noted that the group attended more movies. Third, the doctors rated the health of the choice group as higher than the comparison group. Most striking was an 18-month follow-up that showed twice as many people in the comparison group had died, as opposed to the choice group (Rodin, 1986).

And what of Kitwood's contention that a positive environment can lead to new learning and "rementing"—recovery of lost abilities? There has been research in these areas going back for decades. Research from the 1980s has shown that improving autonomy in nursing homes can improve immune function, overall health, and memory (Rodin, 1986).

On the subject of learning, there is no doubt that people with dementia continue to learn. Individuals with fairly advanced dementia who move to a nursing home can begin to recognize and name care partners who have an ongoing relationship with them. Even people with no verbal skills can show signs of recognition when familiar faces approach. Unfortunately, our biomedical model does not see this for what it represents—the fact that even people with severe dementia can learn and grow.

Sabat (2001) tells of a client, "Dr. B.," who had a hospitalization during a time when his dementia was becoming quite advanced, 8 years after his symptoms began. He had to negotiate a small step when entering the bathroom in his hospital room; this required a special effort, due to his shuffling gait. Initially he would catch his foot on the step, but he soon learned to lift it high enough to clear.

Weeks later, back in the nursing home, Dr. B. continued to reflexively lift his foot when entering the bathroom, even though there was no such step. This demonstrates the concept of implicit memory, which Sabat defines as "a change in a person's behavior as a result of a prior experience, even though the person may not be able to tell you, in words, what he or she has just learned, or even *that* he or she has learned" (p. 290). Bryden (2005) wrote, "I am losing bits of brain, but I am teaching other bits of brain how to do things" (p. 59).

In two Swedish studies (Karlsson, Brane, Melin, Nyth, and Rybo,

1988; Brane, Karlsson, Kohlgren, and Norberg, 1989), the investigators looked at people with dementia in nursing homes for 2 months and 6 months, respectively. While the control groups had the usual care, the other groups were given increased emotional, social, and intellectual stimulation in twice-weekly group sessions, and staff received education about a more engaging approach to care. These studies showed improved cognitive function in the engagement groups, compared to a mild decrease in the controls. (The most significant areas of improvement were in concentration, recent memory, and decreased "absent-mindedness.") The studies also showed spinal fluid evidence of an increase in the levels of certain brain transmitters, suggesting that these chemicals had actually increased as a result of the interactions.

Personal Experience

My own experience shows that the effort to change the culture of care can produce great results in medication reduction. St. John's Home in Rochester, New York, is moving along the transformational path, but we still have far to go. We are a very large home, with 475 elders and nearly 1,000 employees. We still have long hallways, large "units" with nurses' stations, and many double rooms.

In spite of this, we have done better than most in our use of antipsychotic medications. In 2006 and 2007, I had a practice at St. John's that included about 100 people with moderate to severe dementia at any given time. My own audits showed that my antipsychotic use stayed around 7% to 8% during that time, compared to the 40% level seen in most nursing homes in the United States and other industrialized countries. In spite of individual differences, our medical staff as a whole was also well ahead of the norm during that period; our overall use of 14.2% was far below the average antipsychotic use.

As I have moved from full-time practice to an educational role, I plan to roll out a curriculum for care partners based on this book, which will help us to achieve even greater improvements down the road as we continue our transformational journey. Our continued involvement as a registered Eden Alternative home and soon-to-be Green House provider should help ensure our success.

A Trip to Aiken, South Carolina

In addition to our own accomplishments, there are several other organizations around the world that are enjoying success with new ways of looking at dementia. Here is the story of one in particular:

When I attended the 1st International Eden Alternative Conference, held in 2002 in Myrtle Beach, South Carolina, I heard the story of a small home in Aiken, South Carolina. We were told that the Mattie C. Hall Health Care Center had a unit for people with dementia and no one was on an antipsychotic drug. The stories were quite compelling, but as the years passed, I had many questions. Were they preselected to be healthier than the people in most nursing homes? Were they healthier *as a result* of having fewer medications? Was it sustainable over time? If so, how did they do it?

I had a chance to see for myself in 2005. I was scheduled to be in the area, so I took a day to drive down to Aiken. Aiken is a small, rural town, and certainly not a wealthy one. Mattie C. Hall Health Care Center sat on attractive grounds, surrounded by crepe myrtles and an adjoining children's playground. Beyond that, however, there was nothing striking about the layout. A small, one-story nursing home, it nevertheless had a fairly traditional structure to its living area: 40 people with dementia, all receiving Medicaid, with two long halls, a central lounge/dining area, and nurses' station. Many residents slept in double rooms.

The people I saw seemed to be similar to those in other homes. Many had advanced stages of dementia. It was only during a tour with the nurse manager, Pat Bishop, that I realized what was different: the care staff at Mattie C. Hall had transformed their *attitudes* and nowhere was that more apparent than in their leader.

Pat had the type of kind, calm demeanor that was contagious. She showed me around and answered my questions about the people who lived there and how the home functioned. It turned out that, at the moment, they had two people who were on antipsychotic medication. That was 5%—still light-years ahead of most places.

It was clear that the staff reflected the same values in their gentle, loving, and respectful interactions. I asked Pat how they were able to get the part-time medical staff on board with their philosophy of care. Her answer gave me the first of two epiphanies from the visit: "We find that the doctors follow our lead. If we phone them looking for a pill, they will give us one. But if we find other solutions, they will listen and not force pills on us."

My reflection on that answer helped me realize that the best way for me to promote change was to stop spending all of my time simply speaking to the doctors of the world. More important was to teach hands-on care partners the secrets to success and empower them to find the nonpharmacological solutions for the people they know best.

In the end, doctors are as caring as the rest of the world, but they are only as good as the information they receive. When the care staff has the power and ability to use the experiential approach in day-to-day life, the calls for medication will dwindle. My experience with Missy and Bertha (see Chapter 13) the following year reinforced this idea.

The second epiphany occurred when we passed a woman in the lounge who had advanced dementia and was softly calling, "Mary, Mary." Pat stopped for a moment and shared her quiet presence and gentle touch to help the woman feel a momentary connection. As we moved away, I told her that I had learned through the years that "calling out" was one symptom that never responded to pills. Instead of simply agreeing with me, as I had expected, Pat just gave me a quizzical look. Then she said, "I don't see why anyone would think that you have to give someone a pill for something like this!" Here, indeed, was a person who had made the journey to a new understanding of what most of us were still calling *behavior problems*.

The coup de grace from my tour came when I asked Pat about their fall rate. Falls are fairly common in nursing homes—a daily occurrence in many—and I was concerned about the connection with antipsychotic use. She paused and thought for a moment. I assumed she was adding numbers or doing calculations. Finally, she said, "I think . . . Mr. Smith had a fall . . . I believe it was in May." It was now August. I said, "Are you serious? No one else has fallen since then?"

Pat's name came up again recently in San Diego, when Eden board member Sarah Rowan told the story of her husband Joseph's dementia. Joseph's illness was very challenging, and he had "uncontrollable behavior" that forced him to be discharged or removed from two other nursing homes and two day programs. (At one home, Sarah was called and told that Joseph was being belligerent. She arrived to find him naked and handcuffed, with a policeman standing over his bed.)

Sarah heard about the Eden Alternative and Mattie C. Hall, which was several states away, and made a drastic decision. She picked up her belongings and drove her husband to them. When she arrived in the evening, the staff was waiting outside the door to greet them. Her husband was warmly welcomed. Next to the staff stood the home's dog, a Sheltie that reminded Joseph of the dog he had once had. He said to the dog, "What are you doing out here, Mac? Let's go on inside." They did, and he stayed there, content and unmedicated, until his death.

How to Stop a Pill

Many care partners may feel that a person does not need a pill, but they may be uncertain how to proceed. A medical professional will need to be involved, but there are some general guidelines:

1. If a pill has been used for a short time (e.g., during a hospital stay) and there is no sign of distress, it can probably be stopped fairly quickly. If the dose is very low, it may be stopped immediately, but with higher doses, reduce it by half every few days before stopping it completely.

2. If the person is showing excessive sedation or other toxic effects of the pill, it should be stopped quickly. With antipsychotics, this is not usually a problem, but with benzodiazepines (the so-called minor tranquilizers), there can be withdrawal problems.

3. If a person has been on the pill for a long time, and/or you are not sure how much it is needed, the drug should be withdrawn more slowly. Start by reducing the pill by a third to a half and observe for several days. Then keep reducing by this proportion at slow intervals until it is stopped, or until symptoms return.

4. Even if you are fairly sure the person can do without a pill, it may take time for him to adjust to the new environment, or for the care partners to adjust to meet his needs in a more flexible manner. For that reason, pills may sometimes need to be continued for a time before they can be stopped completely.

5. If behavioral expressions increase as the pill is being withdrawn, it does not necessarily mean the pill has to be continued indefinitely. In that case, hold the pill at its present or previous dose, and use the other techniques described in Chapters 11 to 13 to investigate and address underlying needs. The taper can be resumed in the future, when well-being is restored.

It is important to discuss the addictive potential of psychotropic drugs. I say this, not to imply they are addictive to the person with dementia—most are not—but rather that they are often addictive to the physicians and other care partners! This applies to both professional staff and family members.

When I say "addictive," I mean that we get used to feeling that the pill will solve the problem, and we can become anxious and hyperaware of any little change as the dose is reduced. It takes a lot of support and reassurance to keep people invested in medication reduction, as any slight upset can provide justification to try to raise the dose once again. More often than not, these situations are more a case of anxiety on our part than a true need for medication. All of us, doctors included, have been conditioned to rely on these pills, even when the evidence is telling us that they are not effective.

Here is an example of how the process of medication reduction must be paused at times while the care environment is adjusted, but can nevertheless be successful in the long run:

In 2002, Mickey was 94 years old and failing in an assisted living community. When he became more aggressive, an antipsychotic pill was prescribed. He then began to fall and had an overall decline in cognition and function, so he was sent to the hospital. Because he was aggressive toward hospital staff, the pill was increased even further.

When he first came from the hospital to St. John's, Mickey was barely arousable. He was very rigid and appeared to be suffering ill effects from the antipsychotic. The dose was immediately cut in half. Over the next several days, Mickey became more alert but was very confused. He thought he was 32 years old and could not give any recent or past history. As he became more alert, he began to resist personal care, and would often use foul and sexually explicit language. Over the next several days, he was changed to a less-sedating antipsychotic pill, and a mood stabilizer was added, but he continued his tirades. He was also very restless much of the day.

In a care conference, the staff expressed their dissatisfaction with Mickey's placement on their floor. They felt he belonged in a behavioral unit and was not someone they could care for. They asked me for more medication to fix the problem. But so far, the pills had either been ineffective or overly sedating. In spite of their anger and frustration, I offered no change in medication at that time. I agreed to hold the doses steady for the time being, and we discussed his expressions in more detail.

We came up with a long list of interventions, including maximizing freedom of movement and avoiding restraints. We discussed having him avoid crowded group activities and instead engaging him one-to-one during meals and personal care, with an emphasis on kind and positive conversation. We broke his care into smaller increments, spread out over the morning, and discussed using music, reminiscence, and appropriate touch. We solicited more familiar, meaningful belongings from his family and followed his lead in setting his sleep–wake schedule. We searched for more personal history from family and friends.

The group constructed a process to respond to his sexually explicit comments and gestures that would set limits in a humane manner and be consistent across all times of day. We also discussed how personal care can be embarrassing to people and devised ways to preserve modesty. Most of all, I asked the staff to give him more time to get to know us, and for us to get to know him. They were pessimistic about his potential to succeed but agreed to work on it a bit longer.

Over the next few weeks, the phone calls diminished from daily to none at all. At a care conference the following month, I asked how things were going with Mickey. Although his behavioral expressions had not completely disappeared, they had diminished greatly. More important, the staff had learned how to respond to him and no longer viewed him as an unmanageable problem. There was no longer any anger or frustration. They were able to see him with more tenderness and humor, and instead of saying "He doesn't belong here," they were saying, "Oh, you know Mickey—he still has his moments, but we've learned to deal with it."

In this case, the medication was kept going at a relatively safe level while the environment was adapted to Mickey's special needs. Once this state of equilibrium had been reached, it was possible to re-address the removal of these medications, which clearly were adding little or nothing to his care. A couple of months after this plan was put into effect, I again began to taper the drugs—first one and then the other. Mickey got off them completely about 6 months after he arrived, and he remained off them until his peaceful passing, $4\frac{1}{2}$ years later, at the age of 99.

Part of our success came from finding an enlightened approach that eliminated the vast majority of his behavioral expressions. But they did not disappear completely. The other part of our success came from the staff's ability to redefine what was truly a problem, and what was simply an expression by someone with a different perception of the world around him. Doing so allowed them to respond to him as a person deserving of our care and compassion, in a nonjudgmental manner.

Because transformation of care environments takes time, not everyone can be immediately taken off medications and feel calm and engaged. We have had occasions in which a reduction of medication has been unsuccessful. In the vast majority of cases, I still feel we could have succeeded had our environment been more transformed than it was. But a lack of success with some people is no reason to avoid trying to reduce medication in all. Over the years, for every 10 people in whom I have reduced medication doses, perhaps one or two have had to stay on them. However, that still means that eight or nine people are now able to live without the medication; and in those who succeed, the positive results we have seen speak for themselves.

It may seem unrealistic to expect that we can care for people without using any psychotropic drugs for their behavioral expressions. What is clear, however, is that a new approach to dementia can drastically reduce the use of these medications, making them the exception rather than the rule.

We have seen a similar learning curve with the use of physical restraints in nursing homes. Due to the tireless work of pioneers, including Carter Catlett Williams, Lois Evans, and Neville Strumpf, these once-common features of nursing homes are rapidly disappearing. Many nursing homes are now restraint-free; I have not personally ordered a physical restraint in over a decade. Could antipsychotic use in dementia become the "physical restraints of the 21st century"? My hope is that a similar learning curve will lead to the equally rapid removal of these drugs from daily use.

Make no mistake—this is hard work. It takes the combined efforts of many people to transform a model of care, and constant vigilance to prevent the phenomenon of "institutional creep" that attempts to pull us back into the status quo. And yet, the potential benefits are enormous—not just the expected clinical improvements and cost savings (billions in unused antipsychotic pills alone) but the improved well-being of millions of people who live with dementia, their care partners, families, and friends.

There will always be naysayers who will cling to the status quo and complain that such a change is too difficult, too expensive, too risky. In what he calls "the myth of perfection," Bill Thomas (2008) describes the tendency of such people to look for the exception as a means to reject the entire model. I hear this all the time: "Well, it all sounds good, but how about Mrs. X? There's no way you could treat her without an antipsychotic!"

The answer of course is, "You're right—not in the world she is living in today. That's why we have to create a new one for her. Doesn't she, don't we all, deserve it? If there will be 100 million people in the world living with dementia in 40 years, we had better get it right!"

———————————

There is really no better way to end a book espousing an experiential philosophy than with the words of two of those who know the experience best, and who have shared their wisdom with the world—Richard Taylor (2007):

> All I want, all I need, all I ask for is that others, especially my caregivers, be more like me. Not to act like me, but to understand me as I understand myself. I just want others to anticipate my needs and wants. I just want others to try every day to figure me out, to understand me. I just want others to love me as I love them. (p. 218)

and Christine Bryden (2005):

> Our main fear is the "loss of self" associated with dementia. We face an identity crisis. We all believe the toxic lie of dementia that the mind is absent and the body is an empty shell. . . . But we can find a new identity as an emotional being. . . . In our relationships, we can connect at a deeper level. . . . I believe that people with dementia are making an important journey from cognition, through emotion, into spirit. I've begun to realize what really remains throughout this journey is what is really important, and what disappears is what is not important. I think that if society could appreciate this, then people with dementia would be respected and treasured. (pp. 156, 159)

REFERENCES

Abbott, J. H. (1981). *In the belly of the beast: Letters from prison.* New York: Random House.

Administration on Aging. (2008). *A Profile of Older Americans. 2008.* Retrieved from Administration on Aging Web site: http://www.aoa.gov/AoAroot/Aging_Statistics/Profile/Index.aspx.

Alzheimer's Association. (2009). In *2009 Alzheimer's Disease Facts and Figures.* Retrieved May 1, 2009, from Alzheimer's Association Web site: http://alz.org/national/documents/report_alzfactsfigures2009.pdf.

Alzheimer's Disease International. (2009). Retrieved April 1, 2009, from http://www.alz.co.uk/research/statistics.

Avorn, J., Soumerai, S. B., Everitt, D. E., Ross-Degnan, D., Beers, M. H., Sherman, D., et al. (1992). A randomized trial of a program to reduce the use of psychoactive drugs in nursing homes. *New England Journal of Medicine, 327*(3), 168–173.

Baker, B. (2007). *Old age in a new age: The promise of transformative nursing homes.* Nashville: Vanderbilt University Press.

Ballard, C., Hanney, M. L., Theodoulou, M., Douglas, S., McShane, R., Kossakowski, K., et al. (2009). The dementia antipsychotic withdrawal trial (DART-AD): Long-term follow-up of a randomised placebo-controlled trial. *Lancet Neurology, 8*(2), 152–157.

Ballard, C., Margallo-Lana, M., Juszczak, E., Douglas, S., Swann, A., Thomas, A., et al. (2005). Quetiapine and rivastigmine and cognitive decline in Alzheimer's disease: Randomised double blind placebo controlled trial. *British Medical Journal, 330,* 874–878.

Ballard, C., Margallo-Lana, M., Theodoulou, M., Douglas, S., McShane, R., Jacoby, R., et al. (2008, April 1). *A randomised, blinded, placebo-controlled trial in dementia patients continuing or stopping neuroleptics (The DART-AD Trial).* Retrieved May 1, 2009, from PloS Medicine Web site: http://www.plosmedicine.org/article/info:doi/10.1371/journal.pmed.0050076.

Baltes, M. M. (1988). The etiology and maintenance of dependence in the elderly: Three phases of operant research. *Behavior Therapy, 19,* 301–319.

Barrick, A. L., Rader, J., Hoeffer, B., Sloane, P. D., & Biddle, S. (2001). *Bathing without a battle: Person-directed care of individuals with dementia* (2nd ed.). New York: Springer. Retrieved from http://www.bathingwithoutabattle.unc.edu.

Basting, A. (2003). Dare to imagine: Exploring the creative potential of people with Alzheimer's disease and related dementia. In J. Ronch & J. Goldfield (Eds.), *Mental wellness and aging: Strength-based approaches* (pp. 353–367). Baltimore: Health Professions Press.

Bell, V., & Troxel, D. (1997). *The best friends approach to Alzheimer's care.* Baltimore: Health Professions Press.

Blanchard, K., Carlos, J. C., & Randolph, A. (1999). *The 3 keys to empowerment: Release the power within people for astonishing results.* San Francisco: Berrett-Koehler Publishers.

Brane, G., Karlsson, I., Kohlgren, M., & Norberg, A. (1989). Integrity-promoting care of demented nursing home patients: Psychological and biochemical changes. *International Journal of Geriatric Psychiatry, 4,* 165–172.

Brawley, E., & Noell-Waggoner, E. (2008). *Lighting: Partner in quality care environments.*

Retrieved November 1, 2008, from Pioneer Network Web site: http://www.pioneer-network.net/Data/Documents/BrawleyNoell-WagonerLightingPaper.pdf.

Breggin, P. R. (1997). *Brain disabling treatments in psychiatry: Drugs, electroshock and the role of the FDA.* New York: Springer.

Briesacher, B. A., Limcangco, R., Simoni-Wastila, L., Doshi, J. A., Levens, S. R., Shea, D. G., et al. (2005). The quality of antipsychotic drug prescribing in nursing homes. *Archives of Internal Medicine, 165,* 1280–1285.

Brody, E. (1971). Excess disabilities of mentally impaired aged: Impact of individualized treatment. *Gerontologist, 25,* 124–133.

Bronskill, S. E., Anderson, G. M., Sykora, K., Wodchis, W. P., Gill, S., Shulman, K. I., et al. (2004). Neuroleptic drug therapy in older adults newly admitted to nursing homes: Incidence, dose and specialist contact. *Journal of the American Geriatrics Society, 52*(5), 749–755.

Brooker, D. (2007). *Person-centered dementia care: Making services better.* Philadelphia: Jessica Kingsley Publishers.

Bryden, C. (2005). *Dancing with dementia: My story of living positively with dementia.* Philadelphia: Jessica Kingsley Publishers.

Burger, S. (1992). Eliminating inappropriate use of chemical restraints (special section). *Quality Care Advocate, 7,* i–iv.

Carboni, J. (1990). Homelessness among the institutionalized elderly. *Journal of Gerontological Nursing, 16*(7), 3–37.

Carr, D. C. (2005). Changing the culture of aging: A social capital framework for gerontology. *Hallym International Journal of Aging, 7*(2), 81–93.

Carstensen, L. L., Pasupathi, M., Mayr, U., & Nesselroade, J. R. (2000). Emotional experience in everyday life across the adult life span. *Journal of Personality and Social Psychology, 79*(4), 644–655.

Chen, C., Sloane, P., & Dalton, T. (2003, January 23). *Lighting and circadian rhythms and sleep in older adults.* Electric Power Research Institute (Monograph #1007708, http://my.epri.com/portal/server.pt?).

Cheston, R., & Bender, M. (1999). *Understanding dementia: The man with the worried eyes.* Philadelphia: Jessica Kingsley Publishers.

Clapin-French, E. (1986). Sleep patterns of aged people in long-term care facilities. *Journal of Advanced Nursing, 11,* 57–66.

Cohen, U., & Day, K. (1993). *Contemporary environments for people with dementia.* Baltimore: Johns Hopkins University Press.

Cohen-Mansfield, J. (2001). Nonpharmacologic interventions for inappropriate behaviors in dementia. *American Journal of Geriatric Psychiatry, 9*(4), 361–381.

Cohen-Mansfield, J. (2003). Nonpharmacologic interventions for psychotic symptoms in dementia. *Journal of Geriatric Psychiatry and Neurology, 16*(4), 219–224.

Cohen-Mansfield, J. (2005). Non-pharmacological interventions for persons with dementia. *Alzheimer's Care Quarterly, 6*(2), 129–145.

Cohen-Mansfield, J. (2005, May). *Current research in cure and care for agitation.* Paper presented at the meeting of the Alzheimer's Australia National Conference. Retrieved April 28, 2009, from http://www.alzheimers.org.au/content.cfm?infopage id=4150.

Cohen-Mansfield, J., & Bester, A. (2006). Flexibility as a management principle in dementia care: The Adards example. *Gerontologist 46*(4): 540–544.

Cohen-Mansfield, J., Lipson, S., Werner, P., Billig, N., Taylor, L., & Woosley, R. (1999). Withdrawal of haloperidol, thioridazine and lorazepam in the nursing home: A controlled, double-blind study. *Archives of Internal Medicine, 159,* 1733–1740.

Cohen-Mansfield, J., Marx, M. S., & Rosenthal, A. S. (1989). A description of agitation in a nursing home. *Journal of Gerontology, 44*(3), M77–M84.

Cohen-Mansfield, J., & Mintzer, J. E. (2005). Time for change: The role of non-pharmacological interventions in treating behavior problems in nursing home residents with dementia. *Alzheimer's Disease and Associated Disorders, 19*(1), 37–40.

Danish Medicines Agency. (2005, April 26). *Consumption of antipsychotics in Denmark among the elderly.* Retrieved from Danish Medicines Agency Web site: http://www.dkma.dk/1024/visUKLSArtikel.asp?artikelID=5969.

De Deyn, P. P., Rabheru, K., Rasmussen, A., Bocksberger, J. P., Dautzenberg, P. L. J., Eriksson, S., et al. (1999). A randomized trial of risperidone, placebo, and haloperidol for behavioral symptoms of dementia. *Neurology, 53,* 946–955.

Deremeik, J., Broman, A. T., Friedman, D., West, S. K., Massof, R., Park, W., et al. (2007). Low vision rehabilitation in a nursing home population: The SEEING Study. *Journal of Visual Impairment and Blindness, 101,* 701–714.

Dijkstra, K., Bourgeois, M., Youmans, G., & Hancock, A. (2006). Implications of an advice-giving and teacher role on language production in adults with dementia. *Gerontologist, 46,* 357–366.

Ertel, K. A., Glymour, M. M., & Berkman, L. F. (2008). Effects of social integration on preserving memory function in a nationally representative US elderly population. *American Journal of Public Health, 98*(7), 1215–1220.

Feil, N., & de Klerk-Rubin, V. (2002). *The validation breakthrough: Simple techniques for communicating with people with Alzheimer's-type dementia* (2nd ed., Rev.). Baltimore: Health Professions Press.

Fossey, J., Ballard, C., Juszczak, E., James, I., Alder, N., Jacoby, R., et al. (2006). Effect of enhanced psychosocial care on antipsychotic use in nursing home residents with severe dementia: Cluster randomised trial. *British Medical Journal, 332,* 756–761.

Fox, N. (2007). *The journey of a lifetime: Leadership pathways to culture change in long-term care.* Milwaukee: Action Pact, Inc.

Fox, N., Norton, L., Rashap, A. W., Angelelli, J., Tellis-Nyack, V., Grant, L. A., et al. (2005). Well-being: Beyond quality of life (unpublished, obtainable from info@edenalt.org).

Frankl, V. (1959). *Man's search for meaning.* New York: Simon & Schuster.

Fratiglioni, L., Wang, H. X., Ericsson, K., Maytan, M., & Winblad, B. (2000). Influence of social network on occurrence of dementia: A community-based longitudinal study. *Lancet, 255,* 1315–1319.

Fritsch, T., Kwak, J., Grant, S., Lang, J., Montgomery, R. R., & Basting, A. D. (2009). Impact of TimeSlips, a creative expression intervention program, on nursing home residents with dementia and their caregivers. *Gerontologist, 49,* 117–127.

Gill, S. S., Bronskill, S. E., Normand, S. T., Anderson, G. M., Sykora, K., Lam, K., et al. (2007). Antipsychotic drug use and mortality in older adults with dementia. *Annals of Internal Medicine, 146*(11), 775–786.

Gill, S. S., Rochon, P. A., Herrmann, N., Lee, P. E., Sykora, K., Gunraj, N., et al. (2005). Atypical antipsychotic drugs and risk of ischaemic stroke: Population based retrospective cohort study. *British Medical Journal, 330,* 445–448.

Gladwell, M. (2002). *The tipping point: How little things can make a big difference.* Newport Beach, CA: Back Bay Books.

Goldman, D. (2008, September 23). A "revolution" for senior care. *Brighton-Pittsford Post,* p. 1A.

Gottlieb-Tanaka, D., Lee, H., & Graf, P. (Eds.). (2008). *Creative-Expressive Abilities Assessment.* Vancouver, BC: ArtScience Press.

Hawkley, L. C., Masi, C. M., Berry, J. D., & Cacioppo, J. T. (2006). Loneliness is a unique predictor of age-related differences in systolic blood pressure. *Psychology and Aging, 21*, 152–164.

Hirose, S. (2003). The causes of underdiagnosing akathisia. *Schizophrenia Bulletin, 29*(3), 547–558.

Holden, U., & Woods, R. T. (1995). *Positive approaches to dementia care.* New York: Churchill Livingstone.

Horton, J. A. (2005). *A model leadership curriculum for managers of an Eden Alternative nursing home.* Unpublished master's thesis, University of New Hampshire–Durham.

IMS Health. (2006, February). Retrieved January 2, 2007, from IMS Health Web site: http://www.imshealth.com/ims/portal/front/articleC/0,2777,6599_18731_7705 6778,00.html.

Innes, A. (2003). *Dementia care mapping: Applications across cultures.* Baltimore: Health Professions Press.

Jennifer. (2008, March 10). Retrieved February 11, 2009, from Revolution Health Web site: http://revolutionhealth.com/groups/ambush-of-being-bipolar/discussions/topic/a7c21880-2c1c-48cc-9d40-4ec2b4c59d45.

Jones, D. (1999). *Everyday Creativity* (motion picture). (Available from Star Thrower Distribution, 26 East Exchange St., Suite 600, St. Paul, MN 55101.)

Jones, G. (1985). Validation therapy: A companion to reality orientation. *The Canadian Nurse, 81*(3), 20–23.

Kales, H. C., Valenstein, M., Kim, H. M., McCarthy, J. F., Ganoczy, D., Cunningham, F., et al. (2007). Mortality risk in patients with dementia treated with antipsychotics versus other psychiatric medications. *American Journal of Psychiatry, 164*, 1568–1576.

Kane, R. A., Lum, T. Y., Cutler, L. J., Degenholz, H. B., & Yu, T. (2007). Resident outcomes in small-house nursing homes: A longitudinal evaluation of the initial Green House program. *Journal of the American Geriatrics Society, 55*(6), 832–839.

Karlawish, J. (2006). Alzheimer's disease: Clinical trials and the logic of clinical purpose. *New England Journal of Medicine, 355*(15), 1604–1606.

Karlsson, I., Brane, G., Melin, E., Nyth, A. L., & Rybo, E. (1988). Effects of environmental stimulation on biochemical and psychological variables in dementia. *Acta Psychologica Scandinavica, 77*, 207–213.

Katz, I. R., Jeste, D. V., Mintzer, J. E., Clyde, C., Napolitano, J., & Brecher, M. (1999). Comparison of risperidone and placebo for psychosis and behavioral disturbances associated with dementia: A randomized, double-blind trial. *Journal of Clinical Psychiatry, 60*(2), 107–115.

Kay, G. G., Abou-Donia, M. B., Messer, W. J., Murphy, D. C., Tsao, J. W., & Ouslander, J. G. (2005). Antimuscarinic drugs for overactive bladder and their potential effects on cognitive function in older adults. *Journal of the American Geriatrics Society, 53*(12), 2195–2201.

Kitwood, T. (1997). *Dementia reconsidered: The person comes first.* New York: Open University Press.

Kitwood, T., & Bredin, K. (1992). Towards a theory of dementia care: Personhood and well-being. *Aging and Society, 12*, 269–287.

Knol, W., Van Marum, R. J., Jansen, P. A. F., Souverein, P. C., Schobben, A. F. A. M., & Egberts, A. C. (2008). Antipsychotic drug use and the risk of pneumonia in elderly people. *Journal of the American Geriatrics Society, 56*(4), 661–666.

Kouzes, J. M. (2000, October 10). *Link me to your leader.* Retrieved May 1, 2009, from Tom Peters Company Web site: http://www.TomPeters.com.

Kuhn, D., & Verity, J. (2008). *The art of dementia care.* Clifton Park, NY: Thomson Delmar Learning.

Laing, R. D. (1965). *The divided self*. Baltimore: Penguin Books.

Langer, E. J., & Rodin, J. (1976). The effects of choice and enhanced personal responsibility for the aged: A field experiment in an institutional setting. *Journal of Personality and Social Psychology, 34*, 191–198.

Lee, H. (2007). *The impact of the "Spark of Life" program on the personal and emotional wellbeing of people with dementia: Carers' and families' perceptions*. Unpublished master's dissertation, Curtin University of Technology, Perth, Western Australia.

Leonard, R., Tinetti, M. E., Allore, H. G., & Drickamer, M. A. (2006). Potentially modifiable resident characteristics that are associated with physical or verbal aggression among nursing home residents with dementia. *Archives of Internal Medicine, 166*, 1295–1300.

Levitin, D. J. (2006). *This is your brain on music: The science of a human obsession*. New York: Dutton.

Lowe, J. (1998). *Oprah Winfrey speaks: Insights from the world's most influential voice*. Hoboken, NJ: Wiley.

Margallo-Lana, M., Swann, A., O'Brien, J., Fairbairn, A., Reichelt, K., Potkins, D., et al. (2001). Prevalence and pharmacological management of behavioural and psychiatric symptoms amongst dementia sufferers living in care environments. *International Journal of Geriatric Psychiatry, 16*(1), 39–44.

Maslow, A. H. (1943). A theory of human motivation. *Psychological Review, 50*, 370–396.

McGowin, D. F. (1993). *Living in the labyrinth: A personal journey through the maze of Alzheimer's*. Forest Knolls, CA: Elder Books.

McLean, A. (2007). Dementia care as a moral enterprise: A call for the return to the sanctity of lived time. *Alzheimer's Care Today, 8*(4), 360–372.

McShane, R., Keene, J., Gedling, K., Fairburn, C., Jacoby, R., & Hope, T. (1997). Do antipsychotic drugs hasten cognitive decline in dementia? Prospective study with necropsy follow up. *British Medical Journal, 314*, 266–270.

Mehrabian, A. (1981). *Silent messages: Implicit communication of emotions and attitudes* (2nd ed.). Belmont, CA: Wadsworth.

Mintzer, M. Z., Frey, J. M., Yingling, J. E., & Griffiths, R. R. (1997). Triazolam and zolpidem: A comparison of their psychomotor, cognitive, and subjective effects in healthy volunteers. *Behavioral Pharmacology, 8*(6–7), 561–574.

Mintzer, M. Z., & Griffiths, R. R. (1999). Triazolam and zolpidem: Effects on human memory and attentional processes. *Psychopharmacology, 144*(1), 8–19.

Nilsson, J., Rana, A. K., & Kabir, Z. N. (2006). Social capital and quality of life in old age: Results from a cross-sectional study in rural Bangladesh. *Journal of Aging and Health, 18*(3), 419–434.

Otmani, S., Demazieres, A., Staner, C., Jacob, N., Nir, T., Zisapel, N., et al. (2008). Effects of prolonged-release melatonin, zolpidem, and their combination on psychomotor functions, memory recall, and driving skills in healthy middle aged and elderly volunteers. *Human Psychopharmacology, 23*(8), 693–705.

Pearce, N. (2007). *Inside Alzheimer's: How to hear and honor connections with a person who has dementia*. Taylors, SC: Forrason Press.

Perrin, T. (1997). Occupational need in severe dementia: A descriptive study. *Journal of Advanced Geriatric Nursing, 25*(5), 934–941.

Phair, L., & Good, V. (1998). *Dementia: A positive approach*. London: Whurr Publishers Ltd.

Phillips, C. D. (2001). Measuring and assuring quality care in nursing homes. In L. Noelker & Z. Harel (Eds.), *Linking quality of long-term care and quality of life* (pp. 162–181). New York: Springer.

Pollack, C. E., & von dem Knesebeck, O. (2004). Social capital and health among the aged: Comparisons between the United States and Germany. *Health and Place, 10*(4), 383–391.

Porsteinsson, A. P., Tariot, P. N., Erb, R., & Gaile, S. (1997). An open trial of valproate for agitation in geriatric neuropsychiatric disorders. *American Journal of Geriatric Psychiatry, 5*(4), 344–351.

Proust, M. (1929). *The Captive.* New York: Random House, pp. 348–349.

Psychiatric News. (2006, May 19). *New brands may help offset generic competition.* Retrieved January 3, 2007, from Psychiatric News Web site: http://pn.psychiatryonline.org/cgi/content/full/41/10/25-a.

Rader, J., & Tornquist, E. M. (1995). *Individualized dementia care: Creative, compassionate approaches.* New York: Springer.

Rapoport, M., Mamdani, M., Shulman, K., Herrmann, N., & Rochon, P. (2005). Antipsychotic use in the elderly: Shifting trends and increasing costs. *International Journal of Geriatric Psychiatry, 20*(8), 749–753.

Ray, W. A., Taylor, J. A., Meador, K. G., Lichtenstein, M. J., Griffin, M. R., Fought, R., et al. (1993). Reducing antipsychotic drug use in nursing homes: A controlled trial of provider education. *Archives of Internal Medicine, 153,* 713–721.

Ready, R. E., & Ott, B. R. (2003). Quality of life measures for dementia. *Health and Quality of Life Outcomes, 1,* 1–9.

Reisberg, B., Borenstein, M. D., Salob, S. P., Ferris, S. H., Franssen, E., & Georgotas, A. (1987). Behavioral symptoms in Alzheimer's disease: Phenomenology and treatment. *Journal of Clinical Psychiatry, 48* (suppl.), 9–15.

Rodin, J. (1986). Aging and health: Effects of the sense of control. *Science, 233,* 1271–1276.

Rosebrook, V. (2002). Intergenerational connections enhance the personal/social development of young children. *International Journal of Early Childhood, 34*(2), 30–41.

Rosebrook, V. (2007). Intergenerational personal/social skills development study. *Childhood Education, 83*(3), 162P–162R.

Rovner, B. W., Steele, C. D., Shmuely, Y., & Folstein, M. F. (1996). A randomized trial of dementia care in nursing homes. *Journal of the American Geriatrics Society, 44*(1), 7–13.

Rush, C. R., & Griffiths, R. R. (1996). Zolpidem, triazolam and temazepam: Behavior and subject-rated effects in normal volunteers. *Journal of Clinical Psychopharmacology, 16*(2), 146–157.

Sabat, S. R. (2001). *The experience of Alzheimer's disease: Life through a tangled veil.* Malden, MA: Blackwell Publishers.

Sachdev, P. (1995). The development of the concept of akathisia: A historical overview. *Schizophrenia Research, 16*(1), 33–45.

Sato, Y., Metoki, N., Iwamoto, J., & Satoh, K. (2003). Amelioration of osteoporosis and hypovitaminosis D by sunlight exposure in stroke patients. *Neurology, 61,* 338–342.

Schneider, L. S., Dagerman, K. S., & Insel, P. (2005). Risk of death with atypical antipsychotic treatment for dementia. *Journal of the American Medical Association, 294*(15), 1934–1943.

Schneider, L. S., Tariot, P. N., Dagerman, K. S., Davis, S. M., Hsiao, J. K., Ismail, M. S., et al. (2006). Effectiveness of atypical antipsychotic drugs in patients with Alzheimer's disease. *New England Journal of Medicine, 355*(15), 1525–1538.

Sheafor, B. W., & Horejsi, C. R. (2006). *Techniques and guidelines for social work practice* (7th ed.). London: Allyn & Bacon.

Sink, K. M., Holden, K. F., & Yaffe, K. (2005). Pharmacological treatment of neuropsychiatric symptoms of dementia: A review of the evidence. *Journal of the American Medical Association, 293*(5), 596–608.

Sloane, P. D., Mitchell, C. M., Calkins, M., & Zimmerman, S. I. (2000). Lighting and noise levels in Alzheimer's disease special care units. *Research and Practice in Alzheimer's Disease, 4,* 241–249.

Snowden, J., Day, S., & Baker, W. (2005). Why and how antipsychotic drugs are used in 40 Sydney nursing homes. *International Journal of Geriatric Psychiatry, 20*(12), 1146–1152.

Snowden, M., & Roy-Byrne, P. (1998). Mental illness and nursing home reform: OBRA-87 ten years later. *Psychiatric Services, 49,* 229–233.

Stehman, J., Strachan, G. I., Glenner, J. A., Glenner, G. G., & Neubauer, J. K. (1996). Activities based on positive use of perseveration. In *Handbook of dementia care* (pp. H-IV 18–19). Baltimore: Johns Hopkins University Press.

Svarstad, B. L., Mount, J. K., & Bigelow, W. (2001). Variations in the treatment culture of nursing homes and responses to regulations to reduce drug use. *Psychiatric Services, 52*(5), 666–672.

Taylor, R. (2007). *Alzheimer's from the inside out.* Baltimore: Health Professions Press.

Thomas, W. H. (2004). *What are old people for? How elders will save the world.* Acton, MA: VanderWyk & Burnham.

Thomas, W. H. (2006). *In the arms of elders: A parable of wise leadership and community building.* Acton, MA: VanderWyk & Burnham.

Thomas, W. H. (2008). Conference call/webinar with Eden Alternative Mentors, 2/08.

Turner, E. H., Matthews, A. M., Linardatos, E., Tell, R. A., & Rosenthal, R. (2008). Selective publication of antidepressant trials and its influence on apparent efficacy. *New England Journal of Medicine, 358*(3), 252–260.

Tutu, D. M. (1999). *No future without forgiveness.* New York: Doubleday.

Uman, G. C. (1997). Where's Gertrude? *Journal of the American Geriatrics Society, 45*(8), 1025–1026.

Van Reekum, R., Clarke, D., Conn, D., Herrmann, N., Eryavec, G., Cohen, T., et al. (2002). A randomized, placebo-controlled trial of the discontinuation of long-term antipsychotics in dementia. *International Psychogeriatrics, 14*(2), 197–210.

Verity, J. (2002). The Spark of Life program for people with dementia. (Paper presented at the Eden Alternative 1st International Conference. Myrtle Beach, SC, November, 2002.)

Verity, J., & Lee, H. (2008). *Spark of Life club program handbook: A whole new world of dementia care.* Mooroolbark, Victoria, Australia: Dementia Care Australia Pty. Ltd.

Whitehouse, P. J., & George, D. (2008). *The myth of Alzheimer's: What you aren't being told about today's most dreaded diagnosis.* New York: St. Martin's Press.

Wikipedia (2009, March 30). Existential crisis. Retrieved April 1, 2009, from http://en.wikipedia.org/wiki/Existential_crisis.

Williams, K. N., Herman, R., Gajewski, B., & Wilson, K. (2009). Elderspeak communication: Impact on dementia care. *Journal of Alzheimer's Disease and Other Dementias, 24*(1), 11–20.

Wooltorton, E. (2002). Risperidone (Risperdal): Increased rate of cerebrovascular events in dementia trials. *Canadian Medical Association Journal, 167,* 1269–1270.

Wooltorton, E. (2004). Olanzapine (Zyprexa): Increased incidence of cerebrovascular events in dementia trials. *Canadian Medical Association Journal, 170,* 1395.

Zeigler, M. (2008, September 12). Day care operator going to prison. *Democrat and Chronicle,* pp. A1, A6.

RESOURCES

Alzheimer's Association U.S.: http://www.alz.org.

Alzheimer's Disease International: http://www.alz.co.uk.

Eden Alternative: 14500 RR 12, Suite 2, Wimberley, TX 78676. 512-847-6061. http://www.edenalt.org.

Eden at Home: http://www.edenalt.org/eden-at-home/index.html. Contact Laura Beck at 607-351-3082, or LBeck@edenalt.org.

The Green House Project-NCB Capital Impact: 2011 Crystal City Drive, Suite 800, Arlington, VA 22202. 703-647-2313. http://www.ncbcapitalimpact.org/thegreen house.

It's Never 2 Late: 7302 S. Alton Way, Suite 1, Centennial, CO 80112. 303-806-0797. http://www.in2l.com.

Pioneer Network: P.O. Box 18648, Rochester, NY 14618. 585-271-7870. http://www.pioneernetwork.net.

Spark of Life Program: Dementia Care Australia, P.O. Box 378, Mooroolbark, VIC, Australia, 3138. +61 3 9727 2744. http://www.dementiacareaustralia.com.

St. John's Home: 150 Highland Avenue, Rochester, NY 14620. 585-760-1300. http://www.stjohnsliving.org.

INDEX

Note: *f* indicates figures, *t* indicates tables.

Acceptance, 145, 182–183, 185–186
Accusation, 65
Acknowledgment, 145
Active listening, 202–203
Activities
　behavioral expressions and,
　　178–179
　evening routines vs., 194
　music concerts, 118–120
　principles for, 113–118
　spontaneity and variety in, 94
　stories, 115, 117–118
　transformative model and, 233
　See also Meaning in daily life
Adaptive behavior, 192
Adjustment to environments, 26–27
Adulthood, 58–61
Agency staff, eliminating, 95–97
Aggression
　active listening and, 202–203
　akathisia and, 193
　antipsychotics for, xv, 30
　control and, 142, 200, 202, 203
　defusing, 199–201
　environment and, 201–202, 205–206
　language problems and, 155
　noise and, 178
　stories, xv, 36–37, 117–118, 142–143,
　　187–188, 239–240
Aging
Alzheimer's disease as, 12
　being and, 116–117
　in community (*See* Aging in commu-
　　nity)
　hallucinations vs. perception with,
　　218–219
　hearing and, 138
　institutional model on, 54–55
　as pathology, 44
　population increases, 11
　society view of, 57–61, 72, 122
　speech processing and, 149
　vision and lighting with, 89–91

Aging in community
　aging in place dilemma and, 121–122
　deinstitutionalization and, 101–103
　Dementia Units and, 128–130
　global perspective on, 131–132
　Green House Model of, 126–128
　meaning in daily life and, 108
　overview of, 122–125
　stories, 132
　See also Home and community living
Aging in place dilemma, 121–122
Agitation
　antipsychotics for, 30
　approaches to (*See* Agitation and
　　interpersonal approaches)
　in assisted living, 103
　with bathing, 204
　choice in personal care and, 142
　as grief, 112
　language problems and, 155
　needs and, 80
　outpacing and, 65
　reimbursement policies and, 55–56
　restraint avoidance and, 197
　stories, 31–34, 33*f*, 34*f*, 142–143,
　　212–213, 223–224
Agitation and interpersonal approaches
　acceptance and calmness, 185–186
　environmental audit, 176–179
　general approach, 179–181
　medical audit, 171–176
　overview of, 169–170
　psychosocial interventions, 39
　reorient or not, 181–185
　stories, 180, 184–185, 187–188
Aiken (SC), 235–237
Akathisia, 192–193, 201
Alcohol-related dementia, 142–143,
　　154–155
Alertness, 165
Allergic reaction to drugs, 174
Alzheimer's disease
　as aging, 12
　experience of, 84
　resources on, 251
　social sensitivity and, 118

ABOUT THE AUTHOR

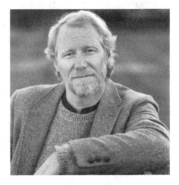

G. Allen Power, M.D., is a board-certified internist and geriatrician and Clinical Associate Professor of Medicine at the University of Rochester, New York. He is also a Fellow of the American College of Physicians–American Society of Internal Medicine. Dr. Power has practiced medicine for 25 years, the last 18 of which have been in long-term care and rehabilitation.

As a Certified Eden Alternative Educator, Dr. Power serves as an Eden Mentor at St. John's Home in Rochester, New York, where he has worked since 2000. He also serves on the board of directors of the Eden Alternative, Inc. His regular contributions to the blog of Dr. William H. Thomas, founder of the Eden Alternative, can be found at www.changingaging.org.

Dr. Power has lectured on geriatric and culture change topics both nationally and internationally. He has been interviewed for print and broadcast media, including BBC *Television*, *The Washington Post*, *The Wall Street Journal*, and WHYY radio, among many others. Dr. Power is also quoted in the book *Old Age in a New Age: The Promise of Transformative Nursing Homes*, by Beth Baker (2007, Vanderbilt University Press).

An accomplished musician and songwriter, Dr. Power's music has been performed on three continents. His song of elder autonomy, "If You Don't Mind," was performed by Peter, Paul and Mary, and Walter Cronkite used his song "I'll Love You Forever" in a 1995 *Discovery Channel* documentary on American families.